ANEMIA IN THE ELDERLY

ANEMIA IN THE ELDERLY

edited by

Lodovico Balducci, MD
Professor of Oncology and Medicine
University of South Florida College of Medicine
Program Leader, Senior Adult Oncology Program
H. Lee Moffitt Cancer Center & Research Institute
Tampa, FL, USA

William B. Ershler, MD
Deputy Clinical Director
National Institute on Aging Intramural Research Program
National Institutes of Health
Harbor Hospital, NM 545
Baltimore, MD, USA

John M. Bennett, MD
Professor of Medicine
Laboratory Medicine and Pathology
James P. Wilmot Cancer Center
University of Rochester Medical Center
Rochester, NY, USA

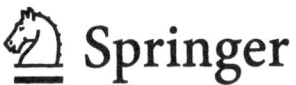 Springer

Lodovico Balducci, MD
University of South Florida College of Medicine
H. Lee Moffitt Cancer Center
Tampa, Florida, USA

William B. Ershler, MD
Clinical Research Branch
Harbor Hospital
Baltimore, Maryland, USA

John M. Bennett, MD
James P. Wilmot Cancer Center
University of Rochester Medical Center
Rochester, New York, USA

Library of Congress Control Number: 2006939207

Printed on acid-free paper.

Hardcover Edition © 2007 Springer Science+Business Media, LLC

ISBN 978-0-387-09791-6   ISBN 978-0-387-49506-4 (eBook)

9 8 7 6 5 4 3 2 1

springer.com

Contents

Contributors

Matti Aapro, MD
Clinique Genolier
Geneve

John W. Adamson, MD
Division of Hematology
Department of Medicine
Medical College of Wisconsin
Medical Services
Blood Center of Wisconsin
Milwaukee, WI

Andrew S. Artz, MD, MS
University of Chicago Pritzker School of Medicine
Department of Medicine
Section of Hematology/Oncology and Section of Geriatrics
Chicago, IL 60637

Lodovico Balducci, MD
Professor of Oncology and Medicine
University of South Florida College of Medicine
Chief Division of Geriatric Oncology
H. Lee Moffitt Cancer Center and Research Institute
Tampa, FL, USA

John M. Bennett, MD
Professor of Medicine, Emeritus
James P. Wilmot Cancer Center
University of Rochester Medical Center
Rochester, NY

Kaaron Benson, MD
Associate Professor of Oncology and Pathology
University of South Florida College of Medicine
Chief Blood Services
H. Lee Moffitt Cancer Center and Research Institute
Tampa, FL, USA

Jeffrey S. Berns, MD
Professor of Medicine and Pediatrics
University of Pennsylvania School of Medicine
Hospital of the University of Pennsylvania
Philadelphia, PA, USA

William B. Ershler, MD
Senior Investigator and Deputy Director
Clinical Research Branch, NIA
Harbor Hospital
National Institute of Health
Baltimore, MD, USA

Bindu Kanapuru, MD
Clinical Research Branch
National Institute on Aging
Baltimore, MD

Ying Liang, PhD
Departments of Internal Medicine and Physiology
Markey Cancer Center
University of Kentucky
Lexington, KY, USA

Alison Miller, PhD
Departments of Internal Medicine and Physiology
Markey Cancer Center
University of Kentucky
Lexington, KY, USA

Erin Oakley, PhD
Departments of Internal Medicine and Physiology
Markey Cancer Center
University of Kentucky
Lexington, KY, USA

Brenda WJH Penninx, PhD
EMGO Institute/Department of Psychiatry
VU University Medical Center
Amsterdam, The Netherlands

Miriam Rodin, MD, PhD
University of Chicago Pritzker School of Medicine
Department of Medicine
Section of Hematology/Oncology and Section of Geriatrics
Chicago, IL 60637

Carol Swiderski, MS
Departments of Internal Medicine and Physiology
Markey Cancer Center
University of Kentucky
Lexington, KY, USA

Gary Van Zant, PhD
Departments of Internal Medicine and Physiology
Markey Cancer Center
University of Kentucky
Lexington, KY, USA

Amanda Waterstrat, PhD
Departments of Internal Medicine and Physiology
Markey Cancer Center
University of Kentucky
Lexington, KY, USA

Chapter 1

Stem Cell Aging: Potential Effects on Health and Mortality

Erin Oakley, Alison Miller, Amanda Waterstrat,
Carol Swiderski, Ying Liang, and Gary Van Zant

Introduction

Aging in a statistical sense is the increasing probability of death with increasing time of an organism's existence (1, 2). Can we extrapolate this to self-regenerating tissues and most particularly to the stem cells that drive the replenishment of lost and damaged cells throughout life? To be succinct, how close is the linkage between the vitality of the stem cell population and organismal longevity? These questions are currently without clear answers and the nature of the linkage, if any, is likely to be complicated, but is nonetheless conceptually compelling. However, in the most straightforward and blunt analysis, limiting numbers of hematopoietic stem cells, for example, resulting in aplastic anemia is an infrequent cause of death (3). Moreover, the hallmark property that distinguishes stem cells from most other somatic cells, their ability to self-replicate, in theory should provide a life-long supply. It was shown many years ago that hematopoietic stem cells could be transplanted into myeloablated recipients and continue to produce large numbers of differentiated blood cells over a time period that greatly exceeded the lifespan of the donor mouse (4). Serial transplants, in which an original bone marrow graft is passaged through a series of recipients, put even greater demands on stem cell proliferation and differentiation and thus demonstrate the tremendous regenerative potential of these cells. However, the number of transplant iterations that may be carried out is limited using marrow from young mice (5, 6), and further reduced if donors are old (6, 7). In fact it is restricted to less than five, depending on mouse strain, and although it has been argued that the limitation is not so much a result of diminished stem cell potential as in the transplantation procedure itself (8), it is now clear that stem cells' regenerative properties diminish during the enforced stress of transplantation and during aging (9–15). Thus, there are growing indications that decrements in stem cell numbers and perhaps more importantly, function, play a role in the aging process. For example, it is well known that age-related decline in the immune system is associated with diminished ability to stave off infection and probably accounts for diminished surveillance and killing of malignant cells (16–21). Whether or not the primary lesion for immune decline resides, at least partially, at the stem cell level is without a definitive answer. For example, in the case of the involution of the thymus, more complicated scenarios, including effects on the thymic epithelium, have been invoked (21). In the context of this volume, the underlying cause of the anemia of the elderly is also not well understood but it too is probably multifactorial, and it remains possible that one of the causes may reside at the level of the hematopoietic stem cell (22, 23). Consistent with this notion is the decades-old observation that the pace of erythropoietic recovery in mice after phlebotomy is protracted in old mice relative to young animals (24). In this review we briefly summarize findings demonstrating several important effects of aging on stem cells. Table 1.1 lists

Table 1.1. Examples of age-related stem cell changes

Stem cell change	Reference
Increased mobilization of stem cells from the bone marrow into the peripheral blood following G-CSF administration	(51)
Diminished homing to bone marrow after transplantation	(11) (32)
Skewed differentiation profile (enhanced myeloid, diminished lymphocytes)	(54) (32)
Decreased self-renewal capacity	(7) (6)
p16^{INK4a} accumulation diminishes self-renewal and response to stress	(6) (86) (87)
Telomere shortening of stem and progenitor cells	(68) (69)
Alteration in population size in humans and mouse that are strain specific	(9) (11) (12) (14)

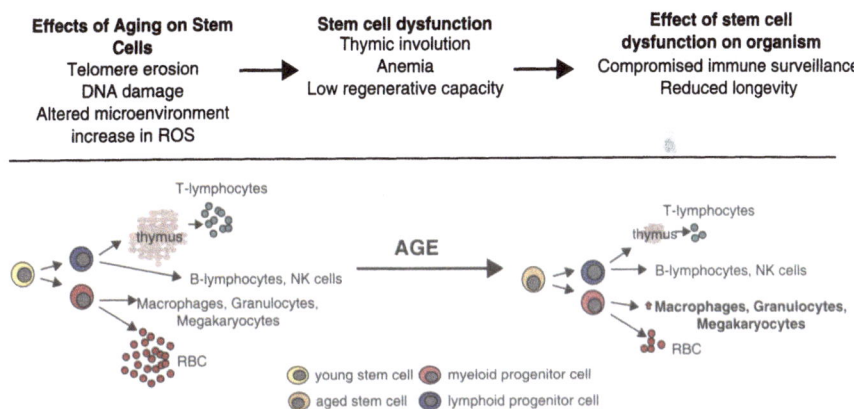

Fig. 1.1. Stem Cell Theory of Aging. At a young age, hematopoietic stem cells possess high regenerative potential and are able to maintain homeostasis of the lymphohematopoietic system. Accumulation of extrinsic insults and intrinsic cellular damage that accompanies aging reduces the regenerative capacity of the stem cell compartment and leads to an imbalance in the production of mature cell types. Reduction of red blood cell numbers and thymic involution may contribute to the decreased immune function observed in older individuals. Simultaneous functional decline in the stem cells of other regenerative tissues may contribute to the aging process, ultimately limiting organismal longevity

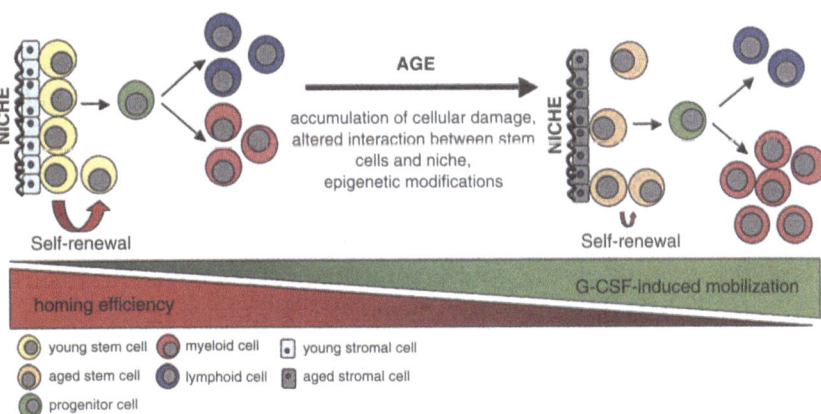

Fig. 1.2. Intrinsic and extrinsic factors in stem cell aging. Age-related changes in the stem cell population and in the cells comprising the microenvironmental stem cell "niche" influence the functional properties of the stem cell. It is thought that a loss in the fidelity of stem cell-microenvironment interactions with age contribute to alterations in homing and G-CSF-induced mobilization. It is likely that microenvironmental changes also contribute to the reduced self-renewal capacity and lineage skewing observed in aged stem cells

examples of the age-related changes on which this review will touch and Fig. 1.1 depicts some of the effects of aging on stem cells that are described in this review.

Interactions Between Stem Cells and Their Microenvironmental "Niche"

Hematopoietic stem cell function, and its change with age, is regulated by a combination of intrinsic (cell-autonomous) and extrinsic influences. Included in the former are genetic and epigenetic influences as well as accumulated damage to cellular components such as mitochondria, membranes, proteins, and chromatin. The effects of age on genome-wide epigenetic changes, principally involving modifications of methylation and acetylation status of DNA and histones, is just starting to be appreciated (25), and is an area of increasing interest and importance in aging research. We and others have recently addressed this issue in reviews highlighting the relationships between epigenetics, aging, and cancer (26, 27, 28). A second frontier of genomic regulation, involving the myriad RNA species transcribed that possess regulatory functions, is at present poorly understood in plants, animals, and humans. The dimension of age at this regulatory level is at this point completely unexplored, but will and should be a burgeoning area of aging research in the future.

Although cell-autonomous responses to aging are undoubtedly important, the effect of aging on the stem cell environment is even less well understood. When hematopoietic stem cells are removed from their native environment in the bone marrow, important extrinsic signals provided by the cells collectively known as the stem "niche" are lost and homeostasis of the stem cell population is disrupted (29). Up to now it has not been possible to reproduce with fidelity the extrinsic signals provided by the "niche," and for this reason it has not been possible to culture and expand stem cell populations ex vivo for potential clinical-scale benefit. Invariably, under even the best of culture conditions, an imbalance develops between self-renewal and differentiation with the latter emphasized at the expense of the former (30). Given the paucity of knowledge regarding the critical elements of the signaling between stem cells and the "niche," it is not surprising that even less is known about the effects of aging on critical cellular and molecular elements of the "niche" (31, 32). The effects of aging on two aspects of stem cells' association with their microenvironmental "niche," homing and mobilization, are discussed below and are summarized in Fig. 1.2. Interestingly, the insight we currently possess has been largely initiated by clinical practice rather than by being driven by basic research. First, the clinical use of bone marrow transplantation to enable high-dose chemotherapy and/or radiation to treat cancer has fostered an appreciation that infused stem cells in the bone marrow graft must find their way to the marrow and properly associate with unoccupied stem cell "niches" in order for engraftment to proceed. Second, drawing on clinical evidence that certain chemotherapeutic agents and, more recently, hematopoietic cytokines, dislodge or "mobilize" stem cells from their "niches" into the circulation has enabled the now standard practice of collecting them by leukapheresis for auto- or allografting rather than by bone marrow harvest.

Effects of Age on Stem Cell Homing

In clinical practice it is difficult to isolate and control for the multiple factors contributing to engraftment following a stem cell transplant. The contribution of the initial event in the process of engraftment, homing of stem cells to the bone marrow, is virtually impossible to assess under clinical conditions. In mice, where it is possible to carefully control for a variety of conditions, it is now recognized that the efficiency of stem cell homing declines as a function of age of the stem cell donor (11, 33). Even under the best of conditions, the fraction of stem cells infused into a myeloablated recipient that can be recovered from the bone marrow within the first day following transplant is less than 10%, and is usually closer to 5% (34–38). There is no reason to believe that the efficiency is significantly higher in humans and the results emphasize the inefficiency of the process rather than the efficient bone marrow-seeking connotation of the term "homing." What is known concerning the effect of age on this process? Only about half as many donor stem cells from old mice (≥ 2 yrs of age) as from young mice can be recovered from the marrow of young recipients (11, 33, 39). Conversely, if stem cells from young adult mice were transplanted into old recipients, the homing efficiency was similarly reduced by about half compared to the fraction of the same stem cell pool recovered from the marrow of young recipients (33). Interestingly, if the ages of both the donor stem cells and the recipient mice are old, the decrements in homing are not synergistic or even additive—homing efficiency is the same whether the donor or the recipient, or both, were old (Liang and Van Zant, unpublished). This result suggests that the effects of age are manifested via a common mechanism necessary for homing and that a defect at either the stem cell or "niche" is sufficient to disrupt homing and lodgement. Therefore, it involves a stem cell-autonomous property and an extrinsic property of the "niche." Although the identity of this pathway is as yet unknown, cell adhesion molecules are the most likely candidates (40–42), since a series of adhesion and motility steps are known to trace the path from the circulation to the marrow "niche" (43). We would be remiss if we did not mention that the properties of the "niche" may change in response to factors such as hematopoietic stress and possibly in response to aging, although the latter is completely unexplored. There is solid evidence supporting the existence of at least two distinctly different "niches"—an endosteal "niche" as well as "niches" supported largely by osteoblasts in the endosteum (44–48). It is not yet clear how or if the two work in concert to meet hematopoietic demands under different physiological conditions. It is conceivable that one type of "niche" may be responsible for promoting the quiescence and lack of proliferation of stem cells, whereas other(s) may promote proliferation and differentiation. Several lines of evidence now support the notion that endosteal "niches" maintain stem cells in a quiescent state (46, 48). Moreover, it is not certain that there are not other types of "niches" that may, under specific conditions, support stem cells. For example, it was shown many years ago that the administration of radioactive strontium (^{89}Sr) to mice caused complete marrow aplasia owing to its concentration in bone and local irradiation of the marrow. The mice survived because life-sustaining hematopoiesis shifted to the spleen, emphasizing that the loss of one type of "niche," endosteal in this experimental model, is not an absolute requisite, and can apparently be compensated for by other "niches," perhaps ones of endothelial-reticular cell origin (45, 49).

Effects of Age on Stem Cell Population Size and Mobilization

In some ways the mobilization of stem cells from their marrow "niche" into the blood circulation must involve a reversal of processes involved in their homing and lodgement following transplantation. Therefore one might expect adhesion molecules, cell motility, and extravasation through the endothelium to be involved, as they are in homing (38). There have been few controlled studies of the effects of age on mobilization. However, because of its widespread use clinically to procure stem cells for transplantation, there is some evidence, mostly anecdotal, that older patients do not mobilize as well for autografting as do younger ones. However, there is also evidence that patients over the age of 60 mobilize equally as well as younger ones (50). The problem with validating this relationship is that the number of confounding variables, including type of malignancy, prior treatment, and co-morbidities, is large and difficult to sort through in meta-analyses. A more promising approach to answering the question of the effect of age on mobilization is to analyze these two parameters in a large group of normal donors mobilized for allografting. To date this type of analysis has not been carried out and the issue of age remains unresolved. Hematologists have long known of the detrimental effect of age on bone marrow cellularity, at least in the commonly sampled sites in the pelvis and sternum (23, 51). Although it is possible that there is a shift in the marrow to other sites such as the vertebrae, ribs, and skull such that overall marrow mass is unaffected by age, this seems highly unlikely. Rather, total hematopoietic mass probably decreases with age with the reduction most pronounced in the very old. It therefore may follow that mobilization may be less effective in the elderly simply because there is less there to mobilize. We have measured the fraction of marrow cells from individuals of a wide age range, and without disease involving any known hematologic function. Iliac crest aspirates showed a steady decline in the fraction of marrow cells that were CD34+, and a regression analysis of almost 50 individuals' marrow showed that almost one quarter (24%) of the variation in CD34+ percentage could be attributed to age (Fig. 1.3). We have also shown in the mouse that the effect of age on hematopoietic stem cell number is highly strain-specific. In DBA/2 mice, as we found with the size of the CD34+ cell population in humans, there is a decline in stem cell number in old age (14). In contrast, in C57BL/6 mice stem cell number increases steadily with age and shows no evidence of decline even out to nearly 3 years of age (11, 14). The effect of age on stem cell mobilization in these two mouse strains might then provide insight into the effect of size of the stem cell pool on mobilization efficiency. Unfortunately, this type of study has been carried out only in the C57BL/6

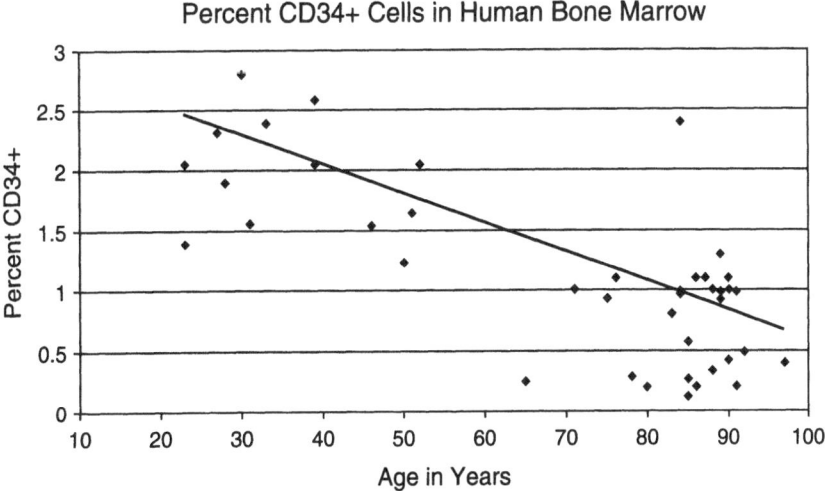

Fig. 1.3. Decline in the percent of CD34+ stem and progenitor cells in human bone marrow with age

strain and it was found that mobilization efficiency increased in old age, commensurate with the overall size of the stem cell population (52). Although the effect of age on mobilization in DBA/2 mice has not been tested, a strain comparison has been carried out in young animals (53). Young C57BL/6 mice were found to mobilize less efficiently than DBA/2 mice as well as other strains. Young DBA/2 mice possess a larger stem cell pool than C57BL/6 mice which may be construed as support for the notion that mobilization efficiency is simply related to the size of the pool to draw upon. However, the fact that there was not a good correlation between stem cell pool size and mobilization efficiency when a larger group of mouse strains was compared, points up the complexity of the mobilization process and the likelihood of other genetic differences contributing to the variation, not the least of which may be strain-specific variation in the response to the mobilizing cytokine G-CSF.

Skewed Differentiation Lineages with Age

Perhaps owing to the overall decline of the immune system during aging briefly discussed above in the Introduction, stem cell transplantation studies have repeatedly shown that engraftment of the immune system is diminished and/or delayed in the face of the enhanced production of myeloid cells, particularly granulocytes and monocytes/macrophages (33, 54, 55). It is worth repeating that during the engraftment process, stem cell function is the net result of intrinsic and extrinsic influences. Cell-autonomous influences, discussed above, include genetic and epigenetic alterations as a function of age, whereas extrinsic influences are manifested via cytokines and other humoral influences but perhaps most importantly through incompletely understood close-range interactions with cells comprising the stem cell "niche" (56) in which stem cells reside. An example of a stem cell-intrinsic change affecting lymphopoiesis is the finding that human CD34+ cells show impaired ability to generate T-cells in culture relative to a similar population from young donors (18). On the extrinsic side of the equation, it has been shown that murine bone marrow stromal cells from old donors, both *in vivo* and *in vitro*, demonstrate an impaired capacity to support B-lymphopoiesis (32, 57). Thus, in old age a mechanism or mechanisms involving both intrinsic and extrinsic levels of regulation, acting individually or in concert, skew stem and progenitor cell differentiation away from lymphopoiesis and toward myelopoiesis (see Figs. 1.1 and 1.2). In the context of this volume, it is similarly appealing to ascribe at least part of the anemia of aging to a lineage profile skewing that to some extent sacrifices erythropoiesis in favor of myelopoiesis.

Telomeres and Stem Cell Aging

After it was first shown that shortening telomere length limited the replicative lifespan of fibroblasts in vitro, and that the resulting senescence could be prevented by enforced expression of telomerase (58, 59), attention turned to this mechanism's potential role in stem cell aging (60, 61). Despite the fact that hematopoietic stem cells, unlike some other cell types, synthesize the holoenzyme telomerase that ameliorates telomere erosion (62), it has been found that human and mouse stem cell telomeres shorten appreciably as a result of replicative stress (63–68). However, the physiological role of telomere length in aging was thrown into question by the finding that in telomerase knockout mice (TERC$^{-/-}$), effects were not seen during the lifetime of first generation animals. However, after several generations of breeding *TERC$^{-/-}$* animals multiple pathologies emerged and, as expected, the first organs to show demonstrable effects were rapidly proliferating tissues such as the bone marrow (69, 71). As a result of unprotected chromosome ends, fusions and other abnormalities resulted in genomic instability followed by tumor formation (71, 72), events that were reversible by enforced telomerase expression (73). Events preceding these catastrophic genomic rearrangements, and which prevented most cells from reaching a malignant state, included cell cycle arrest, senescence and/or apoptosis (74, 75). The fact that telomeres in humans are much shorter than those in mice suggest that some of the telomere-related events found in the murine model may not be applicable for at least some aspects of human telomere study. More than a decade after these seminal studies, it is not clear whether or not diminished telomere length is a cause or an effect of aging, or merely a correlate. This is partly due to the growing understanding of the telomere as a complex chromatin structure rather than simple tandem repeats of primary DNA sequence (TTAGGG in humans). Telomeres have emerged as important binding sites for several important proteins that impart a stable structure to chromosome ends and which in many cases are involved in cellular damage response pathways. Thus, a close relationship exists between telomeres and the cellular mechanisms involved in the detection and correction of cellular damage, or the elimination of damaged cells (75) as depicted in Fig. 1.4.

The Role of Damage–Response Pathways in Stem Cell Aging

If one accepts the premise that stem cell depletion contributes to aging, inhibition of checkpoints that regulate cellular damage by shunting such cells into pathways ending in apoptosis or senescence may preserve stem

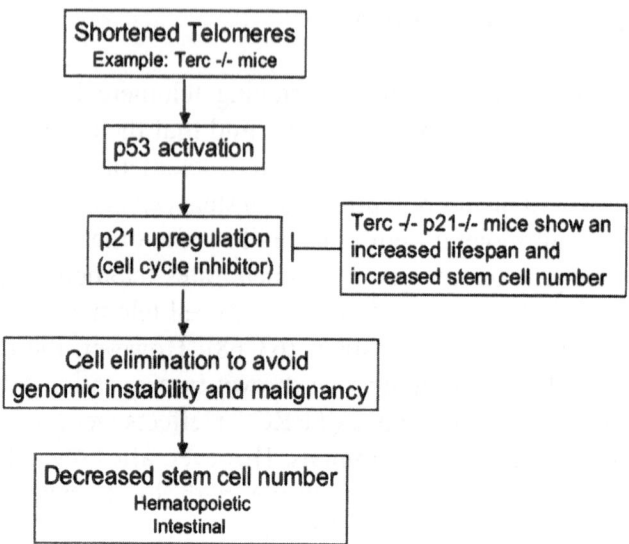

Fig. 1.4. Homeostatic balance between stem cell replication and carcinogenesis. The balance between malignancy and stem cell frequency is tightly regulated by cell cycle checkpoints and DNA damage sensors. This pathway demonstrates the upregulation of p21 in response to critically short telomeres resulting in the cell elimination in order to prevent tumorigenesis. However, if p21 is unable to respond, the outcome is an increase in lifespan and an increase in stem cell frequency

cell numbers at the risk of increased tumorigenesis. For example, p21, encoded by *Cdkn1a*, a cell cycle inhibitor and downstream target of p53, is upregulated in response to short telomeres, consistent with it being important in averting catastrophic genomic rearrangements via processes that eliminate cells (74, 77). In the context of telomeres and aging, a recent study examined the combined effects of *Terc* and *Cdkn1a* deletion. The absence of p21 in fourth generation (G4) *Terc*$^{-/-}$ mice, with critically short telomeres, prolonged their lifespan and improved stem cell function in the hematopoietic system and intestinal epithelium (78). Surprisingly, it did so without an acceleration of tumorigenesis. The fact that p21 deletion did not extend lifespan to that found in G4 *Terc*$^{-/+}$ mice, demonstrates that both p21-dependent and p21-independent mechanisms limit longevity in the context of telomere dysfunction (78).

Fifty years ago, Denham Harman posited and championed what is now called the free radical theory of aging (79). Long-lived cells such as stem cells run the risk of accumulating debilitating damage from a lifetime of normal metabolism and exposure to toxins and cellular stressors (Fig. 1.5). However, until recently, the mechanisms by which reactive oxygen species (ROS) impinge on and are responded to by stem cells has been murky.

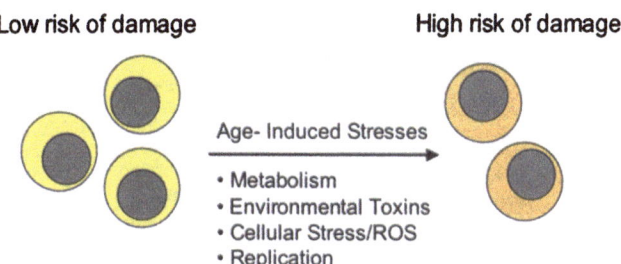

Fig. 1.5. Common sources of stress in aging hematopoietic stem cells that can accumulate, resulting in cellular damage

Elucidation of the role in stem cells of the ATM (Ataxia Telangiectasia Mutated) damage–response pathway has begun to clear up the picture. To interrelate telomere regulation with cellular damage responses, it should be noted that one of the cardinal roles of ATM is in telomere regulation (80). In $Atm^{-/-}$ mice, not only do telomeres dysfunction but cellular oxidant levels rise and it was found that the hematopoietic stem cell population was diminished resulting in aplasia and severe anemia in mice only 6 months old (81, 82). Treatment of $Atm^{-/-}$ mice with the hydrogen peroxide scavenger N-acetyl-cysteine rescued the stem cell aplasia and restored self-renewal via mechanisms independent from the role of ATM in maintaining telomere stability (81). In a recently published extension of these studies, Ito and colleagues showed that oxidative stress in stem cells, but not progenitor cells, activated the p38 MAPK pathway, a relatively general damage control pathway responding to diverse cellular insults (83). This pathway was constitutively activated in $Atm^{-/-}$ mice and was associated with heightened stem cell proliferation. Inhibition of the p38 MAPK pathway reversed stem cell aplasia by returning the bulk of stem cells to a quiescent state. To relate these findings to aging, the authors simulated stem cell aging by serial transplant experiments in wild-type mice. With each transplant not only did the levels of ROS increase in purified stem cells, but p38 MAPK pathway activity increased in concert (83). Thus, stem cells may be depleted during natural aging by an entrained series of events beginning with the accumulation of ROS, subsequent activation of p38, and an increased stem cell cycling but not self-renewal. Since in other cell types increased proliferation is associated with increased cellular ROS (84, 85), a positive feedback loop may similarly be established that enforces the demise of the population. These recent findings are outlined in scenarios depicted in Fig. 1.6.

Recent evidence demonstrates that this may occur not only through the p38 pathway but via the p16 ^{INK4A}-retinoblastoma (RB) activation of protein kinase C (86). Evidence supporting this arm of the cellular damage control

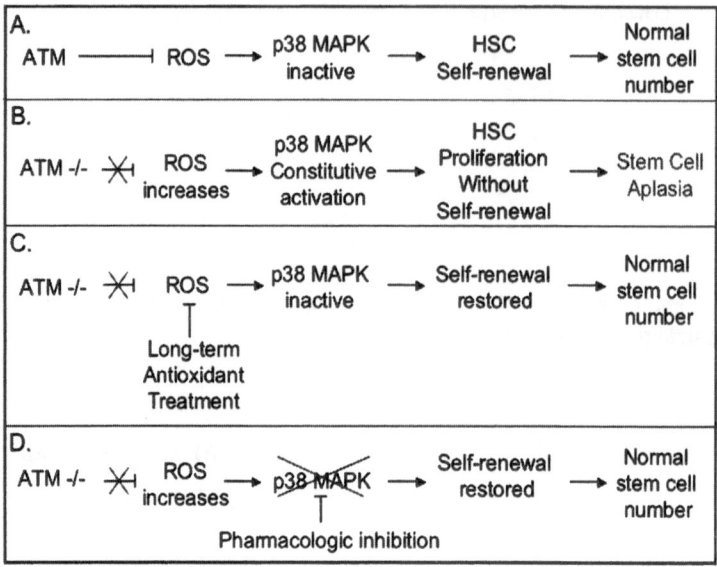

Fig. 1.6. The ATM pathway effects stem cell number. (**A**) The normal function of the ATM pathway yields a normal stem cell number. Here, ATM detects the levels of ROS. When ROS levels reach a critical amount, p38 MAPK is activated, resulting in stem cell self-renewal and proper maintenance of the stem cell pool. (**B**) Mice lacking ATM cannot control the levels of ROS, leading to an increase in oxidative stress. This increase causes constitutive activation of p38 MAPK and excessive stem cell proliferation resulting in differentiation rather than self-renewal. This depletion of the stem cell pool manifests in the whole animal as stem cell aplasia. (**C**) Long-term treatment with antioxidants can deter the constitutive activation of p38 MAPK seen in the ATM knockout mice. With this intervention, the stem cell pool is maintained at normal levels. (**D**) Pharmacologic inhibition of p38 MAPK is another method of restoring normal stem cell proliferation rates and maintaining the stem cell pool in ATM knockout mice. This is not surprising since p38 inhibitors are often incorporated into aplastic anemia therapies

pathway is outlined below and summarized in Fig. 1.7. The *p16^INK4A* cyclin-dependent kinase inhibitor has been shown to enforce G1 cell cycle arrest by activating the RB tumor suppressor which subsequently induces irreversible cellular senescence. In a recent series of papers the role the p16 ^{INK4A}-RB pathway has been brought to the fore in the biology of stem cell aging, not only in the hematopoietic system but in pancreatic islets and in neural stem cells as well (6, 87, 88). In all three regenerative systems, p16 ^{INK4A} rose in stem cells during aging. In the hematopoietic system the increase in p16 ^{INK4A} was found only in the most primitive stem cell population, and not in any of their immediate progeny (6). In *p16 $^{INK4A-/-}$* mice the size of the hematopoietic stem cell population was similar to that of wild-type animals and stem cells from the two strains had equal abilities to reconstitute irradiated recipients. However, after aging 14–24 months, the

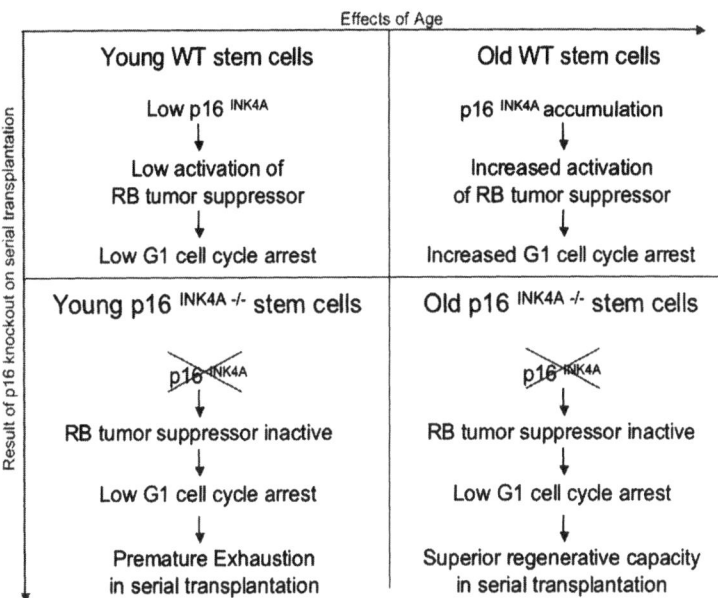

Fig. 1.7. The effects of age on the p16 INK4A pathway. The levels of *p16 INK4A* are low in the primitive hematopoietic stem cells of young mice. Thus, there are low activation levels of the RB tumor suppressor leading to few cells in cell cycle arrest (low senescence). In the primitive hematopoietic stem cells of old mice, the levels of p16 INK4A are high, leading to an increase in RB activation and an increase in the number of cells in G1 cell cycle arrest (high senescence). In p16 INK4A knockout mice subjected to serial transplantation the effects of the gene deletion on the stem cell pool were dramatic. Young cells lacking p16 INK4A were unable to activate the RB pathway to decrease cell cycling and maintain levels of stem cell self-renewal. With the stress of serial transplantation, these mice demonstrated premature exhaustion compared to the wild-type young mice. The old mice also lacked p16 INK4A and therefore could not activate the RB tumor suppressor pathway. Accordingly, they demonstrate low levels of G1 cell cycle arrest. Thus, the cells have increased cell cycling compared to their wild-type counterparts and are able to maintain superior regenerative capacity during serial transplantation

knockout mice had a significantly larger stem cell population with a larger fraction proliferating and were better able to engraft in a transplant setting. Surprisingly, when subjected to serial transplantation, stem cells from young *p16 INK4A−/−* mice showed premature exhaustion compared to age-matched wild-type controls. However, when the same serial transplantation comparison was made using old donor animals, the opposite was true: stem cells from old *p16* knockout mice had superior regenerative capacity (6). Thus p16 INK4A has age-specific effects on hematopoietic stem cell repopulation as has been shown in other populations (89–91). Prevention of the age-related increase of p16 INK4A in stem cells clearly had significant advantages in terms of both numbers and repopulating function. However, the p16 [INK4A]-deficient animals are cancer-prone and have reduced lifespans as a result (92). As pointed out in a commentary to these three papers, the capacity of stem cells for regeneration must be balanced against the probabilities of tumorigenesis (91). While the p16 [INK4A]-RB pathway may limit stem cell numbers through senescence and apoptosis, it acts as a tumor suppressor by eliminating pre-cancerous cells and thus extending a healthy lifespan.

References

1. Hayflick, L. (1998) How and why we age. *Exp Gerontol* 33, 639–653
2. Kirkwood, T. B. L. (1998) Biological theories of aging: An overview. *Aging Clin Exp Res* V, 144–146
3. Rando, T. A. (2006) Stem cells, ageing and the quest for immortality. *Nature* 441, 1080–1086
4. Harrison, D. E. (1972) Normal function of transplanted mouse erythrocyte precursors for 21 months beyond donor life spans. *Nature New Biol* 237, 220–222
5. Siminovitch, L., Till, J. E., and McCulloch, E. A. (1964) Decline in colony-forming ability of marrow cells subjected to serial transplantation into irradiated mice. *J Cell Comp Physiol* 64, 23–31
6. Janzen, V., Forkert, R., Fleming, H. E., Saito, Y., Waring, M. T., Dombkowski, D. M., Cheng, T., DePinho, R. A., Sharpless, N. E., and Scadden, D. T. (2006) Stem-cell ageing modified by the cyclin-dependent kinase inhibitor p16INK4a. *Nature* 443, 421–426
7. Ogden, D. A., and Micklem, H. S. (1976) The fate of serially transplanted bone marrow cell populations from young and old donors. *Transplantation* 22, 287–293
8. Harrison, D. E., Astle, C. M., and Delaittre, J. A. (1978) Loss of proliferative capacity in immunohemopoietic stem cells is caused by serial transplantation rather than aging. *J Exp Med* 147, 1526–1531
9. Chen, J., Astle, B. A., and Harrison, D. E. (1999) Development and aging of primitive hematopoietic stem cells in BALB/cBy mice. *Exp Hematol* 27, 928–935
10. Harrison, D. E. (1983) Long-term erythropoietic repopulating ability of old, young, and fetal stem cells. *J Exp Med* 157, 1496–1504
11. Morrison, S. J., Wandycz, A. M., Akashi, K., Globerson, A., and Weissman, I. L. (1996) The aging of hematopoietic stem cells. *Nat Med* 2, 1011–1016
12. Sudo, K., Ema, H., Morita, Y., and Nakauchi, H. (2000) Age-associated characteristics of murine hematopoietic stem cells. *J Exp Med* 192, 1273–1280
13. de Haan, G., Nijhof, W., and VanZant, G. (1997) Mouse strain-dependent changes in frequency and proliferation of hematopoietic stem cells during aging: Correlation between lifespan and cycling activity. *Blood* 89, 1543–1550
14. de Haan, G., and Van Zant, G. (1999) Dynamic changes in mouse hematopoietic stem cell numbers during aging. *Blood* 93, 3294–3301
15. Marley, S. B., Lewis, J. L., Davidson, R. J., Roberts, I. A. G., Dokal, I., Goldman, J. M., and Gordon, M. Y. (1999) Evidence for a continuous decline in haemopoietic cell function from birth: application to evaluating bone marrow failure in children. *Br J Haematol* 106, 162–166
16. Globerson, A., and Effros, R. B. (2000) Ageing of lymphocytes and lymphocytes in the aged. *Immunol Today* 21, 515–521
17. Miller, R. A. (1996) The aging immune system: primer and prospectus. *Science* 273, 70–74

18. Offner, F., Kerre, T., DeSmedt, M., and Plum, J. (1999) Bone marrow CD34+ cells generate fewer T cells in vitro with increasing age and following chemotherapy. *Br J Haematol* 104, 801–808

19. Effros, R. B. (2001) Ageing and the immune system. *Novartis Found Symp* 235, 130–139; discussion 139–145, 146–139

20. Aspinall, R. (2000) Longevity and the immune response. *Biogerontology* 1, 273–278

21. Min, H., Montecino-Rodriguez, E., and Dorshkind, K. (2005) Effects of aging on early B- and T-cell development. *Immunol Rev* 205, 7–17

22. Lipschitz, D. A., Mitchell, C. O., and Thompson, C. (1981) The anemia of senescence. *Am J Hematol* 11, 47–54

23. Lipschitz, D. A., Udupa, K. B., Milton, K. Y., and Thompson, C. O. (1984) Effect of age on hematopoiesis in man. *Blood* 63, 502–509

24. Harrison, D. E. (1975) Defective erythropoietic responses of aged mice not improved by young marrow. *J Gerontol* 30, 286–288

25. Fraga, M. F., Ballestar, E., Paz, M. F., Ropero, S., Setien, F., Ballestar, M. L., Heine-Suner, D., Cigudosa, J. C., Urioste, M., Benitez, J., Boix-Chornet, M., Sanchez-Aguilera, A., Ling, C., Carlsson, E., Poulsen, P., Vaag, A., Stephan, Z., Spector, T. D., Wu, Y. Z., Plass, C., and Esteller, M. (2005) Epigenetic differences arise during the lifetime of monozygotic twins. *Proc Natl Acad Sci USA* 102, 10604–10609

26. Feinberg, A. P., Ohlsson, R., and Henikoff, S. (2006) The epigenetic progenitor origin of human cancer. *Nat Rev Genet* 7, 21–33

27. Callinan, P. A., and Feinberg, A. P. (2006) The emerging science of epigenomics. *Hum Mol Genet* 15(Spec No 1), R95–R101

28. Oakley, E., and Van Zant, G. (2007) Unraveling the complex regulation of stem cells: Implications for aging and cancer. *Leukemia* 21, 612–621

29. Schofield, R., Lord, B. I., Kyffin, S., and Gilbert, C. W. (1980) Self-maintenance capacity of CFU-S. *J Cell Physiol* 103, 355–362

30. Tisdale, J. F., Hanazono, Y., Sellers, S. E., Agricola, B. A., Metzger, M. E., Donahue, R. E., and Dunbar, C. E. (1998) Ex vivo expansion of genetically marked rhesus peripheral blood progenitor cells results in diminished long-term repopulating ability. *Blood* 92, 1131–1141

31. Chertkov, J. L., and Gurevitch, O. A. (1981) Age-related changes in hemopoietic microenvironment. Enhanced growth of hemopoietic stroma and weakened genetic resistance of hemopoietic cells in old mice. *Exp Gerontol* 16, 195–198

32. Stephan, R. P., Reilly, C. R., and Witte, P. L. (1998) Impaired ability of bone marrow stromal cells to support B-lymphopoiesis with age. *Blood* 91, 75–88

33. Liang, Y., Van Zant, G., and Szilvassy, S. J. (2005) Effects of aging on the homing and engraftment of murine hematopoietic stem and progenitor cells. *Blood* 106, 1479–1487

34. Szilvassy, S. J., Ragland, P. L., Miller, C. L., and Eaves, C. J. (2003) The marrow homing efficiency of murine hematopoietic stem cells remains constant during ontogeny. *Exp Hematol* 31, 331–338

35. Szilvassy, S. J., Meyerrose, T. E., Ragland, P. L., and Grimes, B. (2001) Differential homing and engraftment properties of hematopoietic progenitor cells from murine bone marrow, mobilized peripheral blood, and fetal liver. *Blood* 98, 2108–2115

36. Szilvassy, S. J., Meyerrose, T. E., Ragland, P. L., and Grimes, B. (2001) Homing and engraftment defects in ex vivo expanded murine hematopoietic cells are associated with downregulation of beta1 integrin. *Exp Hematol* 29, 1494–1502

37. Hendrikx, P. J., Martens, C. M., Hagenbeek, A., Keij, J. F., and Visser, J. W. (1996) Homing of fluorescently labeled murine hematopoietic stem cells. *Exp Hematol* 24, 129–140

38. Papayannopoulou, T., and Craddock, C. (1997) Homing and trafficking of hemopoietic progenitor cells. *Acta Haematol* 97(1–2), 97–104

39. Yilmaz, O. H., Kiel, M. J., and Morrison, S. J. (2006) SLAM family markers are conserved among hematopoietic stem cells from old and reconstituted mice and markedly increase their purity. *Blood* 107, 924–930

40. Papayannopoulou, T., Craddock, C., Nakamoto, B., Priestley, G. V., and Wolf, N. S. (1995) The VLA4/VCAM-1 adhesion pathway defines contrasting mechanisms of lodgement of transplanted murine hemopoietic progenitors between bone marrow and spleen. *Proc Natl Acad Sci USA* 92, 9647–9651

41. Williams, D. A., Rios, M., Stephens, C., and Patel, V. P. (1991) Fibronectin and VLA-4 in haematopoietic stem cell-microenvironment interactions. *Nature* 352, 438–441

42. Quesenberry, P. J., Colvin, G., and Abedi, M. (2005) Perspective: fundamental and clinical concepts on stem cell homing and engraftment: a journey to niches and beyond. *Exp Hematol* 33, 9–19

43. Quesenberry, P. J., and Becker, P. S. (1998) Stem cell homing: Rolling, crawling, and nesting. *Proc Natl Acad Sci* 95, 15155–15157

44. Kiel, M. J., Yilmaz, O. H., Iwashita, T., Yilmaz, O. H., Terhorst, C., and Morrison, S. J. (2005) SLAM family receptors distinguish hematopoietic stem and progenitor cells and reveal endothelial niches for stem cells. *Cell* 121, 1109–1121

45. Sugiyama, T., Kohara, H., Noda, M., and Nagasawa, T. (2006) Maintenance of the hematopoietic stem cell pool by CXCL12-CXCR4 chemokine signaling in bone marrow stromal cell niches. *Immunity* 25, 977–988

46. Adams, G. B., Chabner, K. T., Alley, I. R., Olson, D. P., Szczepiorkowski, Z. M., Poznansky, M. C., Kos, C. H., Pollak, M. R., Brown, E. M., and Scadden, D. T. (2006) Stem cell engraftment at the endosteal niche is specified by the calcium-sensing receptor. *Nature* 439, 599–603

47. Nilsson, S. K., Johnston, H. M., and Coverdale, J. A. (2001) Spatial localization of transplanted hemopoietic stem cells: inferences for the localization of stem cell niches. *Blood* 97, 2293–2299

48. Nilsson, S. K., Johnston, H. M., Whitty, G. A., Williams, B., Webb, R. J., Denhardt, D. T., Bertoncello, I., Bendall, L. J., Simmons, P. J., and Haylock, D. N. (2005) Osteopontin, a key component of the hematopoietic stem cell niche and regulator of primitive hematopoietic progenitor cells. *Blood* 106, 1232–1239

49. Kiel, M. J., and Morrison, S. J. (2006) Maintaining hematopoietic stem cells in the vascular niche. *Immunity* 25, 862–864

50. Guba, S. C., Vesole, D. H., Jagannath, S., Bracy, D., Barlogie, B., and Tricot, G. (1997) Peripheral stem cell mobilization and engraftment in patients over age 60. *Bone Marrow Transplant* 20, 1–3

51. Harstock, R. J., Smith, E. B., and Ketter, C. N. (1965) Normal variation with aging of the amount of hematopoietic tissue in bone marrow from anterior iliac crest. *Am J Clin Pathol* 43, 325–333

52. Xing, Z., Ryan, M. A., Daria, D., Nattamai, K. J., Van Zant, G., Wang, L., Zheng, Y., and Geiger, H. (2006) Increased hematopoietic stem cell mobilization in aged mice. *Blood* 108, 2190–2197

53. Roberts, A. W., Foote, S., Alexander, W. S., Scott, C., Robb, L., and Metcalf, D. (1997) Genetic influences determining progenitor cell mobilization and leukocytosis induced by granulocyte colony-stimulating factor. *Blood* 89, 2736–2744

54. Spangrude, G. J., Brooks, D. M., and Tumas, D. B. (1995) Long-term repopulation of irradiated mice with limiting numbers of purified hematopoietic stem cells: in vivo expansion of stem cell phenotype but not function. *Blood* 85, 1006–1016

55. Kim, M., Moon, H. B., and Spangrude, G. J. (2003) Major age-related changes of mouse hematopoietic stem/progenitor cells. *Ann NY Acad Sci* 996, 195–208

56. Schofield, R. (1978) The relationship between the spleen colony-forming cell and the haemopoietic stem cell. *Blood Cells* 4, 7–25

57. Labrie, J. E., 3rd, Sah, A. P., Allman, D. M., Cancro, M. P., and Gerstein, R. M. (2004) Bone marrow microenvironmental changes underlie reduced RAG-mediated recombination and B cell generation in aged mice. *J Exp Med* 200, 411–423

58. Harley, C. B., Futcher, A. B., and Greider, C. W. (1990) Telomeres shorten during ageing of human fibroblasts. *Nature* 345, 458–460

59. Bodnar, A., Ouellette, M., Frolkis, M., Holt, S., Chiu, C.-P., Morin, G., Harley, C., Shay, J., Lichtsteiner, S., and Wright, W. (1998) Extension of life-span by introduction of telomerase into normal human cells. *Science* 279, 349–352

60. Vaziri, H., Dragowska, W., Allsopp, R. C., Thomas, T. E., Harley, C. B., and Lansdorp, P. M. (1994) Evidence for a mitotic clock in human hematopoietic stem cells: loss of telomeric DNA with age. *Proc Natl Acad Sci USA* 91, 9857–9860

61. Brummendorf, T. H., Mak, J., Sabo, K. M., Baerlocher, G. M., Dietz, K., Abkowitz, J. L., and Lansdorp, P. M. (2002) Longitudinal studies of telomere length in feline blood cells: implications for hematopoietic stem cell turnover in vivo. *Exp Hematol* 30, 1147–1152

62. Morrison, S. J., Prowse, K. R., Ho, P., and Weissman, I. L. (1996) Telomerase activity in hematopoietic cells is associated with self-renewal potential. *Immunity* 5, 207–216

63. Rufer, N., Brummendorf, T. H., Chapuis, B., Heig, C., Lansdorp, P. M., and Roosnek, E. (2001) Accelerated telomere shortening in hematological lineages is limited to the first year following stem cell transplantation. *Blood* 97, 575–577

64. Notaro, R., Cimmino, A., Tabarini, D., Rotoli, B., and Luzzatto, L. (1997) In vivo telomere dynamics of human hematopoietic stem cells. *Proc Natl Acad Sci USA* 94, 13782–13785

65. Wynn, R., Cross, M., Hatton, C., Will, A., Lashford, L., Dexter, T., and Testa, N. (1998) Accelerated telomere shortening in young recipients of allogeneic bone-marrow transplants. *Lancet* 351, 178–181

66. Wynn, R., Thornley, I., Freedman, M., and Saunders, E. F. (1999) Telomere shortening in leucocyte subsets of long-term survivors of allogeneic bone marrow transplantation. *Br J Haematol* 105, 997–1001

67. Akiyama, M., Asai, O., Kuraishi, Y., Urashima, M., Hoshi, Y., Sakamaki, H., Yabe, H., Furukawa, T., Yamada, O., Mizoguchi, H., and Yamada, H. (2000) Shortening of telomeres in recipients of both autologous and allogeneic hematopoietic stem cell transplantation. *Bone Marrow Transplant* 25, 441–447

68. Ball, S. E., Gibson, F. M., Rizzo, S., Tooze, J. A., Marsh, J. C. W., and Gordonsmith, E. C. (1998) Progressive telomere shortening in aplastic anemia. *Blood* 91, 3582–3592

69. Blasco, M. A., Lee, H. W., Hande, M. P., Samper, E., Lansdorp, P. M., DePinho, R. A., and Greider, C. W. (1997) Telomere shortening and tumor formation by mouse cells lacking telomerase RNA. *Cell* 91, 25–34

70. Lee, H.-W., Blasco, M., Gottlieb, G., Horner, J., Greider, C., and DePinho, R. (1998) Essential role of mouse telomerase in highly proliferative organs. *Nature* 392, 569–574

71. Rudolph, K. L., Chang, S., Lee, H.-W., Blasco, M., Gottlieb, G. J., Greider, C. W., and DePinho, R. A. (1999) Longevity, stress response, and cancer in aging telomerase-deficient mice. *Cell* 96, 701–712

72. Hande, M. P., Samper, E., Lansdorp, P., and Blasco, M. A. (1999) Telomere length dynamics and chromosomal instability in cells derived from telomerase null mice. *J Cell Biol* 144, 589–601

73. Samper, E., Flores, J. M., and Blasco, M. A. (2001) Restoration of telomerase activity rescues chromosomal instability and premature aging in Terc–/– mice with short telomeres. *EMBO Rep* 2, 800–807

74. Wright, W. E., and Shay, J. W. (1992) The two-stage mechanism controlling cellular senescence and immortalization. *Exp Gerontol* 27, 383–389

75. Lee, H. W., Blasco, M. A., Gottlieb, G. J., Horner, J. W., 2nd, Greider, C. W., and DePinho, R. A. (1998) Essential role of mouse telomerase in highly proliferative organs. *Nature* 392, 569–574

76. Campisi, J. (2005) Senescent cells, tumor suppression, and organismal aging: good citizens, bad neighbors. *Cell* 120, 513–522

77. Allsopp, R. C., Vaziri, H., Patterson, C., Goldstein, S., Younglai, E. V., Futcher, A. B., Greider, C. W., and Harley, C. B. (1992) Telomere length predicts replicative capacity of human fibroblasts. *Proc Natl Acad Sci USA* 89, 10114–10118

78. Choudhury, A., Ju, Z., Djojosubroto, M., Schienke, A., Lechel, A., Schaetzlein, S., Jiang, H., Stepczynska, A., Wang, C., Buer, J., Lee, H.-W., von Zglinicki, T., Ganser, A., Schirmacher, P., Nakauchi, H., and Rudolph, K. (2006) *Cdkn1a* deletion improves stem cell function and lifespan of mice with dysfunctional telomeres without accelerating cancer formation. *Nat Gen,* doi:10.1038/ng1937, 1–7

79. Harman, D. (1956) Aging: a theory based on free radical and radiation chemistry. *J Gerontol* 11, 298–300

80. Wong, K. K., Maser, R. S., Bachoo, R. M., Menon, J., Carrasco, D. R., Gu, Y., Alt, F. W., and DePinho, R. A. (2003) Telomere dysfunction and Atm deficiency compromises organ homeostasis and accelerates ageing. *Nature* 421, 643–648

81. Ito, K., Hirao, A., Arai, F., Matsuoka, S., Takubo, K., Hamaguchi, I., Nomiyama, K., Hosokawa, K., Sakurada, K., Nakagata, N., Ikeda, Y., Mak, T. W., and Suda, T. (2004) Regulation of oxidative stress by ATM is required for self-renewal of haematopoietic stem cells. *Nature* 431, 997–1002

82. Rotman, G., and Shiloh, Y. (1997) Ataxia-telangiectasia: is ATM a sensor of oxidative damage and stress? *Bioessays* 19, 911–917

83. Ito, K., Hirao, A., Arai, F., Takubo, K., Matsuoka, S., Miyamoto, K., Ohmura, M., Naka, K., Hosokawa, K., Ikeda, Y., and Suda, T. (2006) Reactive oxygen species act through p38 MAPK to limit the lifespan of hematopoietic stem cells. *Nat Med* 12, 446–451

84. Irani, K., Xia, Y., Zweier, J. L., Sollott, S. J., Der, C. J., Fearon, E. R., Sundaresan, M., Finkel, T., and Goldschmidt-Clermont, P. J. (1997) Mitogenic signaling mediated by oxidants in Ras-transformed fibroblasts. *Science* 275, 1649–1652

85. Lee, A. C., Fenster, B. E., Ito, H., Takeda, K., Bae, N. S., Hirai, T., Yu, Z. X., Ferrans, V. J., Howard, B. H., and Finkel, T. (1999) Ras proteins induce senescence by altering the intracellular levels of reactive oxygen species. *J Biol Chem* 274, 7936–7940

86. Takahashi, A., Ohtani, N., Yamakoshi, K., Iida, S., Tahara, H., Nakayama, K., Nakayama, K. I., Ide, T., Saya, H., and Hara, E. (2006) Mitogenic signalling and the p16INK4a-Rb pathway cooperate to enforce irreversible cellular senescence. *Nat Cell Biol* 8, 1291–1297

87. Molofsky, A. V., Slutsky, S. G., Joseph, N. M., He, S., Pardal, R., Krishnamurthy, J., Sharpless, N. E., and Morrison, S. J. (2006) Increasing p16INK4a expression decreases forebrain progenitors and neurogenesis during ageing. *Nature* 443, 448–452

88. Krishnamurthy, J., Ramsey, M. R., Ligon, K. L., Torrice, C., Koh, A., Bonner-Weir, S., and Sharpless, N. E. (2006) p16INK4a induces an age-dependent decline in islet regenerative potential. *Nature* 443, 453–457

89. Sharpless, N. E., and DePinho, R. A. (2004) Telomeres, stem cells, senescence, and cancer. *J Clin Invest* 113, 160–168
90. Beausejour, C. M., Krtolica, A., Galimi, F., Narita, M., Lowe, S. W., Yaswen, P., and Campisi, J. (2003) Reversal of human cellular senescence: roles of the p53 and p16 pathways. *Embo J* 22, 4212–4222
91. Beausejour, C. M., and Campisi, J. (2006) Ageing: balancing regeneration and cancer. *Nature* 443, 404–405
92. Kim, W. Y., and Sharpless, N. E. (2006) The regulation of INK4/ARF in cancer and aging. *Cell* 127, 265–275

Chapter 2

Anemia and Aging or Anemia of Aging?

Lodovico Balducci and Matti Aapro

The Western population is aging. Currently, individuals aged 65 and older represent 12% of the US population and by the year 2030 they are expected to represent 20% (1). The segment of the population increasing more rapidly than any other involves individuals over 85, the so called "oldest old." The mean life expectancy of the population was around 60 years in 1900, is currently 80 for women and 76 for man and is expected to rise to 84 and 80, respectively, in 2030 (1).

This epidemic presents medical and social implications. Aging is associated with increased prevalence of chronic diseases, disabilities and functional dependence, that in turn lead to increased demand for medical services as well as for social services and care-giving (2, 3). While aging cannot be prevented, the complications of aging may be preventable or at least delayed. Compression of morbidity may prolong the independence and improve the quality of life of the older aged person and at the same time it may minimize the management-related costs (4, 5).

This chapter explores the interactions of anemia and aging that are of interest for at least three reasons. First, incidence and prevalence of anemia increase with aging (6–8). Second anemia may represent the early sign of an underlying serious disease such as cancer, hypothyroidism or malabsorption (6). Third, anemia itself is associated with increased mortality and disability (7). It is reasonable to expect that prompt and effective management of anemia may help compress the aging-related morbidity.

The causes and the management of anemia in the older aged person will be studied after reviewing the biology of aging.

Biology of Aging and its Clinical Implications

Aging has been defined as loss of entropy and of fractality (9, 10). Loss of entropy implies loss of the functional reserve of multiple organ systems, that involves reduced ability to cope with stress. Loss of fractality entails loss of important physiologic functions. Fractals are repetitive, albeit unpredictable subdivisions of a single unit, such as the bronchi or the neurons. Thus loss of fractality involves decline in the arteriolar alveolar interface in the lung and reduction in the number of neurosynapsis, which in turn leads to reduced ability to perform complex activities. Ultimately, loss of fractality entails decline of one's functional independence, and social and environmental interactions.

Underlying loss of entropy and fractality is a chronic and progressive inflammation that represents the biologic hallmark of aging (11). Seemingly, this inflammation originates from the interaction of individual genetics, diseases, and environment. Increased concentrations of inflammatory cytokines, especially interleukin-6 (IL-6) have been associated with increased mortality, functional dependence, and with a number of geriatric syndromes including dementia and osteoporosis (10, 11). In this perspective, it is not far-fetched to hypothesize that anemia may be both a consequence and a cause of aging (Fig. 2.1). Correction of anemia may break this vicious circle and delay the complications of aging.

Loss of entropy and fractality is reflected in the declining function of several organ systems (12). Of clinical relevance are:

- A progressive decline in glomerular filtration rate (GFR) that is almost universal and may be associated with reduced production of erythrpopoietin;

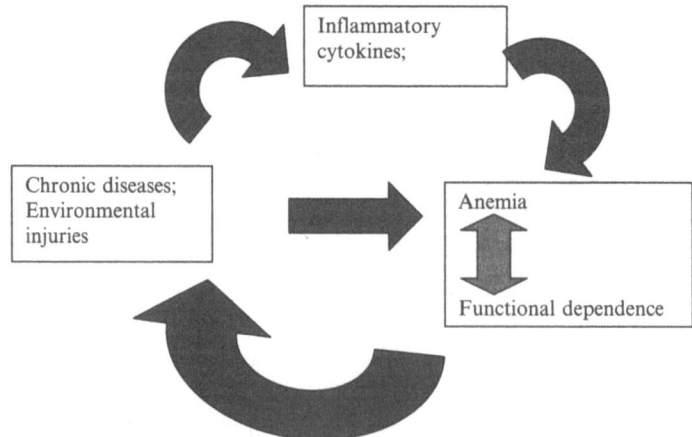

Fig. 2.1. Anemia and aging: a vicious circle

- A progressive decline in the digestion and absorption of nutrients due to reduced gastro-intestinal secretions, gastric motility, splanchnic circulation and absorbing surface. The absorption of iron, that my lead to iron deficiency may be hampered by hepcidine, a glycoprotein synthesized in the liver whose production is stimulated by IL-6 (13). The absorption of B12 may be reduced in older individuals due to inability to digest food bound cobalamaine;
- A number of endocrine changes, including decreased concentration of testosterone and dehydroepiandrotestosterone (DHEA), growth hormone, insulin, and thyroxine, while the concentration of corticosteroids in the circulation may be increased (14);
- Progressive reduction in marrow cellularity, associated with reduced ability to withstand hemopoietic stress (15). This has become particularly evident with cytotoxic chemotherapy of cancer that causes more frequent and severe neutropenia and thrombocytopenia in older individuals.

Aging is universal, albeit highly individualized and is poorly reflected in chronologic age, as it can be seen by the fact that individuals of similar age have different risks of mortality and functional dependence (Fig. 2.2) (16). The management of the older aged person involves an assessment of the physiologic age of each individual. While it is common practice to screen individuals 70 and older for age-related problem, it would be a disservice to consider everybody in this age group as "elderly." Age 70 is just a landmark beyond which the risk of being old increases: by no means it is by itself a sign of old age.

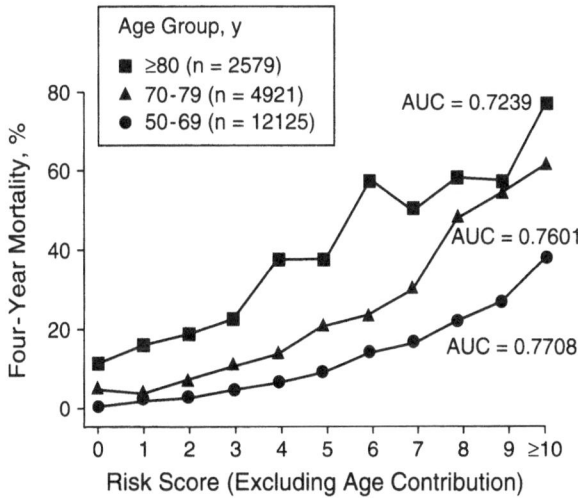

Fig. 2.2. Risk of 4 year mortality based on age and a score computed from function and comorbidity (16)

Clinical Evaluation of Aging

In the absence of reliable measurements of entropy and fractality, the clinical assessment of age relies mainly on the clinical evaluation of the patient. A comprehensive geriatric assessment (CGA) is a time honored assessment of aging and involves the evaluation of function, comorbidy, presence or absence of ageriatric syndromes, as well as of polipharmacy, social support, and nutrition. An example of CGA utilized by the Senior Adult Oncology Program (SAOP) at the H. Lee Moffitt Cancer Center and Research Institute is illustrated in Table 2.1 (17).

In addition to the ADLs and IADLs, the assessment of the advanced activities of daily living (AADL), that is the ability to perform enjoyable activities (such as playing golf or dancing) is also part of the assessment of the functional status (17), as an indirect assessment of one's quality of life.

The comorbid conditions of major interest, because they have been associated with increased risk of mortality include cardiovascular diseases, renal insufficiency, and cancer (16). Comorbidity scales assess both the number and the seriousness of comorbid conditions. Scales of common use include the Charlson scale (17), that is particularly useful in epidemiological studies, and the CIRS-G that proved the most sensitive in our experience (17).

Geriatric syndromes are conditions that are typical, albeit not unique, of aging. Approximately 20% of cancer patients aged 70 and older had some form of early dementia or sub-clinical depression when screened for these conditions (18). Early detection of dementia may allow prompt institution of medications that delay memory loss, and appropriate social arrangements to prevent a person from being hurt. In rare cases, a reversible cause of memory disorder, such as cobalamine deficiency, hypothyroidism, or normal pressure hydrocephalus may be identified (19, 20). Sub-clinical depression is associated with increased mortality in older people (21) and is reversible in the majority of cases. Screening women over 65 for osteoporosis is a recommended intervention, as proper treatment may reverse this condition. There are no clear guidelines for screening man, though they too may experience osteoporosis with aging, especially when hypogonadic (22). Neglect and abuse suggest at least inadequate caregiving, but may also be a sign of deeper problems, including criminal activities in the elder's home. Failure to thrive is a poorly defined but well-recognized condition, in which a person undergoes progressive weight loss and functional decline despite adequate food intake (23). This condition is generally terminal, may involve different causes. Seemingly, inflammatory cytokines are the main mechanism of failure to thrive.

Table 2.1. The CGA at the SAOP: clinical implications

Domain	Assessment	Clinical implication
Functional status	Performance status (PS) Activities of daily living (ADL): • Transferring • Feeding • Grooming • Dressing • Use of the bathroom Instrumental activities of daily living (IADL): • Use of transportations • Use of telephone • Ability to take medications • Financial management • Shopping • Ability to provide to one's nutrition	Dependence in ADL and IADLs: Increased risk of mortality Increased vulnerability to stress Dependence in ADLs: need for a home caregiver Dependence in IADL: need for a caregiver Explore possibility of functional rehabilitation
Comorbidity	Number of comorbid conditions Comorbidity scales	Risk of mortality and vulnerability to stress increases with the number and severity of comorbid conditions Optimal management of diseases may improve patient health and prevent functional decline
Geriatric syndromes	Dementia (screen) Depression (screen) Delirium Falls (screen for risk of falls) Osteoporosis Dizziness Neglect and abuse Failure to thrive	Increased risk of mortality and functional dependence Increased vulnerability to stress Medication may delay dementia, reverse depression and osteoporosis Fall prevention
Nutrition	Assessment of malnutrition and of risk of malnutrition	Malnutrition is associated with increased vulnerability to stress
Polypharmacy	Number of medications Risk of drug interactions	Complications and cost
Social support	Personal resources Social resources	

Approximately 20% of individuals 70 and older have some degree of malnutrition (18), and many more are at risk for malnutrition, due to lack of appetite, depression, isolation, and inadequate access to food. Most of the risk factors for malnutrition are reversible.

The CGA is time consuming and may not be necessary for all individuals who appear healthy and independent. For this purpose a number of screening tests have been proposed to identify individuals in need of more "in depth" assessment. Of these, the five-item screening instrument of the cardiovascular health study (CSH) had gained almost universal acceptance, because it is very simple to perform and has been validated in 8500 individuals followed for an average of 11 years (24) (Table 2.2). This instrument is capable to identify three groups of otherwise independent individuals: fit, pre-frail, and frail, with different risk of mortality, hospitalization, and admission to an assisted living facility.

As aging is associated with a chronic and progressive inflammation, it is reasonable to explore the possibility that the concentration of inflammatory cytokines and other markers of inflammation in the circulation may reflect a person's chronologic age. While definitive studies of the subject have not been produced as yet, Cohen et al. demonstrated that increased concentrations of IL-6 and D-Dimer in the circulation of home-dwelling individuals aged 70 and over were associated with increased risk of mortality and functional decline (25).

Thus, a reasonable approach to a person 70 and older that is independent, may involve the CHS assessment first, followed by a more "in depth" evaluation of individuals who score as pre-frail and frail. The concentration of inflammatory cytokines in the circulation may become important in the near future.

Table 2.2. The CHS assessment

A. Variables of interest
- Involuntary weight loss of ≥10% of the original body weight over 1 year or less;
- Decreased grip strength
- Early exhaustion
- Slow walk
- Difficulty in starting movements.

B. Clinical groups:
- Fit: negative assessment
- Pre-frail: 1–2 abnormal parameters
- Frail: 3 or more abnormal parameters

Frailty and its Implications

The CHS calls pre-frail and frail individuals with one or more abnormalities in the five evaluation parameters. The term frailty has been considered for long time germane to if not synonymous of old age, and it recurs in the geriatric jargon. At a recent consensus conference on frailty (10), agreement was reached on two basic points:

- Frailty implies a condition of increased vulnerability to stress;
- Frailty is a syndrome characterized by sarcopenia, malnutrition, reduced strength and endurance, and reduced neuromuscular adaptability.

Frailty overlaps to some extent with comorbidity and loss of function, but comorbidity and loss of function by themselves cannot account for all cases of frailty.

While the definition and the understanding of frailty is evolving, the practitioner should be aware of the fact that a group of elderly individuals present increased vulnerability to stress, increased risk of functional dependence, and decreased life expectancy. These individuals may be identified by a number of signs, including reduction of sight and hearing, polipharmacy, uncertain gait, episodes of memory loss and of delirium, falls, etc. (26, 27). Identification of frail individuals is important for at least two reasons. The Assessment and Care of Vulnerable Elderly (ACOVE) study clearly demonstrated that management focused on areas of vulnerability may improve the survival and the autonomy of frail individuals (28). Also, any treatment plan for a specific disease involving a frail person must take into account that the benefits of treatment may be lessened by reduced life-expectancy and increased risk of therapeutic complications.

Clearly, the term frailty embraces a wide array of conditions, from that of a person with reduced exercisa endurance to that of a person unable to walk. A so called "frailty index" proposed in 2004 by Mitnitski et al., may provide a quantitative measurement of frailty (29). This index, that is based on the assessment of 70 conditions including function, activities, and disease has been correlated in different patient cohorts with the risk of mortality and hospitalization (29). According to the authors, this index may provide an estimate of a person's physiologic age. While it has been used so far for population studies, the frailty index may become a useful assay of individual life expectancy and functional reserve.

Assessment of Treatment Outcome

In the following discussion, we will explore the effects of anemia on the older aged person and the potential benefits of managing anemia. Together with life prolongation, "compression of morbidity" is a major goal of managing older people (4, 5). This involves delay of the manifestations of disease and preservation of function until the latest times of life.

Preservation of function may be assessed as:

- Functional independence, that implies independence of all ADLs and IADLs essential for living alone;
- Reduction, reversal or delay of impairments, disabilities and handicaps. Impairment involves the progressive loss of a function, such as the movement of a lower extremity; impairment may lead to disability, such as inability to climb stairs; an uncompensated disability is a handicap; for example, inability to climb stairs becomes a handicap if the building does not provide an elevator or an escalator.
- Proves of physical performance, including strength of upper and lower extremities.

Epidemiology and Causes of Anemia in Older Age

The incidence and prevalence of anemia increase with age. The NHANES III study (6) found that the prevalence of anemia was approximately 9.5% in individuals aged 65 and older, increased with age, and it was higher for African-Americans, when compared with Caucasians, non black Hispanic and Asian-Americans. Anemia was more common in older man than in older women, a finding that needs qualification. The NHANES III adopted the definition of anemia of the World Health Organization (WHO), that normal hemoglobin values are ≥12 gm/dl for women and ≥13.0 gm/dl for man. The accuracy of these values has been questioned since the publications of the Woman Health and Aging studies (WHAS), demonstrating that in women 65 and older hemoglobin levels <13.5 gm/dl were associated with increased risk of mortality (30) and of functional impairment (31). If there is no reason to expect that the average hemoglobin levels should be lower in older women than in older men, as suggested by the WHAS, the prevalence of anemia in the NHANES III is similar for both sexes.

The NHANES III data are consistent with the studies of Olmstead county that demonstrated an age-related increase in incidence and prevalence of anemia. The prevalence of anemia was somehow higher in Olmsted county, as this was a survey of the full population, including the sickest and oldest individuals (8). The data are also consistent with the Italian cross-sectional study that showed a prevalence of anemia of 9.2% for individuals aged 65 and over (32). The Italian study showed that the average hemoglobin levels did not change with age, whereas the prevalence of anemia increased with age, suggesting that anemia, even mild anemia, is not a consequence of age by itself. This suggestion has been challenged by a Japanese cohort study, showing that in the absence of any disease or impairment the values of hemoglobin decreased by 0.036 gm/dl/year for women and by 0.04 gm/dl for men between age 70 and 80 (33). Irrespective of whether there is a modest drop in average hemoglobin levels with age, this appears negligible and unable to explain the increased incidence of anemia in the elderly.

The most common causes of anemia in older individuals in the NHANES III and the Olmstead county study are shown in Table 2.2. It is possible that with more investigations a specific cause might have been found for the so called anemias of unknown causes, including early myelodysplasia, and anemia of renal insufficiency, as the GFR declines with age in the majority of cases, and this decline has not been associated with increase in the concentration of serum creatinine (12). A number of studies indicated that the secretion of erythropoietin by the kidney may decrease when the GFR drops below 60 ml/dl (34).

Recent findings are germane to the discussion of the causes of anemia in older individuals:

- Incidence and prevalence of B12 deficiency increase with age (35, 36). The most common cause of B12 deficiency is the inability to digest food B12 due to decreased gastric secretion of hydrochloric acid and of pepsin, and may be responsive to oral crystalline B12. In addition to anemia, B12 deficiency may be a cause of neurologic disorders including dementia, and posterior column lesions.
- Seemingly, the main cause of iron deficiency is chronic bleeding, from cancer, diverticuli, or angiodysplasia. In older age iron deficiency may have other causes, including decreased absorption of iron, due to gastric achylia, and to increased circulating concentrations of hepcidin. Hepcidin prevents the absorption of iron from the duodenum, and is a protein synthesized in the liver, whose production is stimulated by IL-6 (37) A recently recognized cause of iron deficiency is H Pylori gastritis (38).
- In some older individuals the secretion of erythropoietin and the erythropoietic response to erythropoietin may be impaired, as a result of increased circulating concentrations of IL-6 and other inflammatory cytokines (39, 40). In elderly patients from Chianti, Ferrucci et al. demonstrated that increased concentration of inflammatory cytokines in the circulation is associated with increased concentrations of erythropoietin initially, followed by reduced response of erythropoietin to anemia

(Fig. 2.3) (39). Similar findings were reported in a sample of patients from the Baltimore Longitudinal Study by Ershler et al. (40). These studies suggest a biphasic response of erythropoietin to inflammatory cytokines: an initial increased production of erythropoietin even for normal hemoglobin levels, followed by a reduced response of erythropoietin to the drop of hemoglobin concentration. This condition of relative erythropoietin deficiency, similar to relative insulin deficiency in type II diabetes, is exacerbated by increased resistance of erythropoietic progenitors to erythropoietin, also mediated by IL-6, and increased circulating levels of hepcidine, that prevent mobilization of iron from iron stores. Is there a difference between anemia of aging and anemia of chronic inflammation (ACI) (41)? Certainly there is almost complete overlap in the pathogenesis of the two forms of anemia, and aging may be considered a chronic progressive inflammation. At present there is not good reason to distinguish the two entities.

• In the INCHIANTI study Ferrucci et al. found that anemia was associated with low testosterone levels both in men and women and that low testosterone levels predicted the development of anemia in non anemic

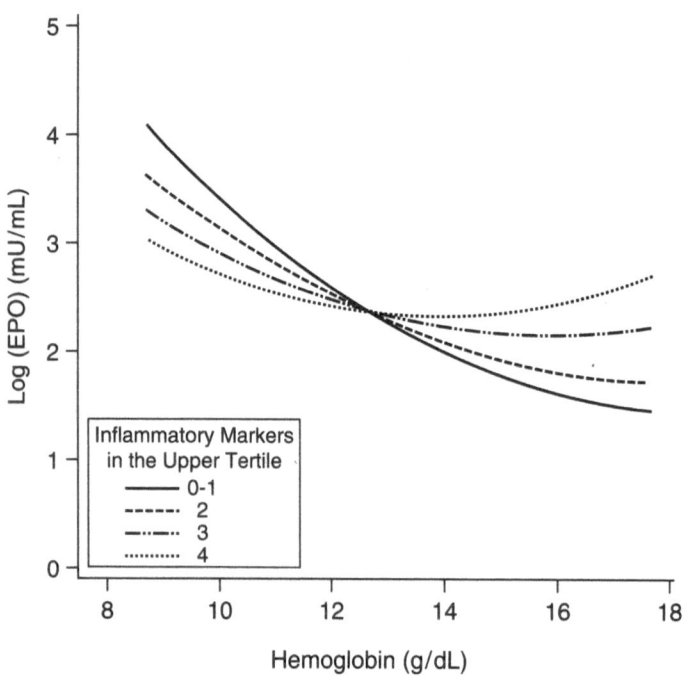

Fig. 2.3. Recommended diagnostic investigations of anemia

individuals over the next 3 years (42). The role of hypogonadism in the development of anemia deserves further exploration especially in view of the current trend to treat older men with testosterone replacement.

- Recent studies show that lenalidomide may induce a complete cytogenetic response in patients with refractory anemia and q (–) cytogenetic abnormalities (43) and may prolong the survival of these patients. Thus, work up for myelodysplasia in older individuals with mild anemia of unknown causes may avert to some extent the mortality and morbidity from this condition. This hypothesis should be tested in randomized controlled studies.

Consequences of Anemia

The clinical consequences of anemia are listed in Table 2.3.

At least seven cohort studies demonstrated that anemia is an independent risk factor for mortality in older individuals (8, 30, 44–48). Of these, the most provocative are the WHAS and the study by Zakai et al. The WHAS reported an increased risk of mortality for hemoglobin levels <13.4 gm/dl home dwelling women aged 65 and over followed for an average of 11 years, and may mandate a revision of the WHO definition of anemia in older women (30). The study by Zakai found that mortality was increased for hemoglobin levels lower than 12.7 gm/dl for women and 13.5 gm/dl for men (47).

Table 2.3. Consequences of anemia

Increased risk of mortality
Increased risk of functional dependence
Increased risk of dementia
Increased risk of delirium
Increased risk of chemotherapy-related toxicity
Increased risk of congestive heart failure and coronary death
Increased risk of falls

Development of functional dependence represents the failure of one of the major goals in the management of older individuals: compression of morbidity. Clearly, functional dependence is one of the most serious consequences of anemia in older individuals (31, 49–51). In the WHAS, the EPESE, and the Chianti studies anemia after age 65 was associated with increased risk of dependence in instrumental activities of daily livings (IADLs) and with mobility impairments. The risk of functional dependence and of mobility impairment was inversely related to the levels of hemoglobin, when these dropped below 13.5 gm/dl. This finding was constant in all studies and suggests that even mild anemia may have serious consequences for the independence of older individuals.

Anemia is associated with increased risk of therapeutic complications from medications and from surgery. Anemia was an independent risk factor for the complications of cytotoxic chemotherapy in at least five studies (52–56). The majority of antineoplastic agents are bound to red blood cells, so that the concentration of free drug in the circulation and the risk of toxicity are increased in the presence of anemia. It is also possible that chronic hypoxia of normal tissue may enhance the susceptibility of these tissues to treatment complications. Seemingly, hypoxia of the brain increases the risk of delirium from medications in older individuals with anemia (57).

The association of chronic anemia and congestive heart failure is well known (58–61). A review of Medicare record showed that individuals 65 and older with myocardial infarction and hematocrit lower than 30% were more likely to die if they did not receive any blood transfusions (62).

Studies in patients with chronic renal failure suggested that anemia might have been a cause of dementia, as the risk of dementia was significantly increased among patients whose anemia had not been corrected with erythropoietin (63). A recent study by Atti et al. demonstrated that the risk of dementia was higher in the presence of anemia among older patients, and anemic individuals with normal mental status were more likely than non-anemia patients of the same age to develop dementia over 5 years (65). Other authors reported increased risk of cognitive dysfunctions in older individuals even with mild anemia (65, 66).

According to a recent study anemia was also associated with increased risk of falls, both in institutions and in the community (67). Falls are a geriatric syndrome, associated with increased mortality and morbidity, including hip fractures.

At this point it should be emphasized that currently there is no proof that correction of mild anemia in older patients will avert the complications of anemia. Anemia of a specific cause of course should be corrected. Correction of ACI with erythropoietic growth factors improves the fatigue of cancer patients, but so far no other benefits of this approach have been demonstrated (68).

Diagnosis and Management of Anemia

Diagnosis of Anemia

As the WHO criteria for the diagnosis of anemia have been challenged in recent studies, it appears reasonable to institute a work up for anemia when hemoglobin levels are lower than 13 gm/dl both in man and women. Seemingly for some individuals, especially woman and African-Americans, hemoglobin levels between 12 and 13 gm/dl are normal, and they should be considered normal if no cause of anemia becomes apparent and the hemoglobin does not drop for one year or longer.

The basic work up of anemia is illustrated in Fig. 2.4. Only rarely a hyper-proliferative anemia may present as chronic anemia. This is the case with micro-angiopathic anemia in individuals with artificial heart valves or severe vascular diseases. Though the mean cellular volume (MCV) may direct the diagnosis, it is prudent to investigate all common causes of anemia in older individuals irrespective of the MCV, as the simultaneous presence of multiple deficiencies may influence the MCV in opposite directions.

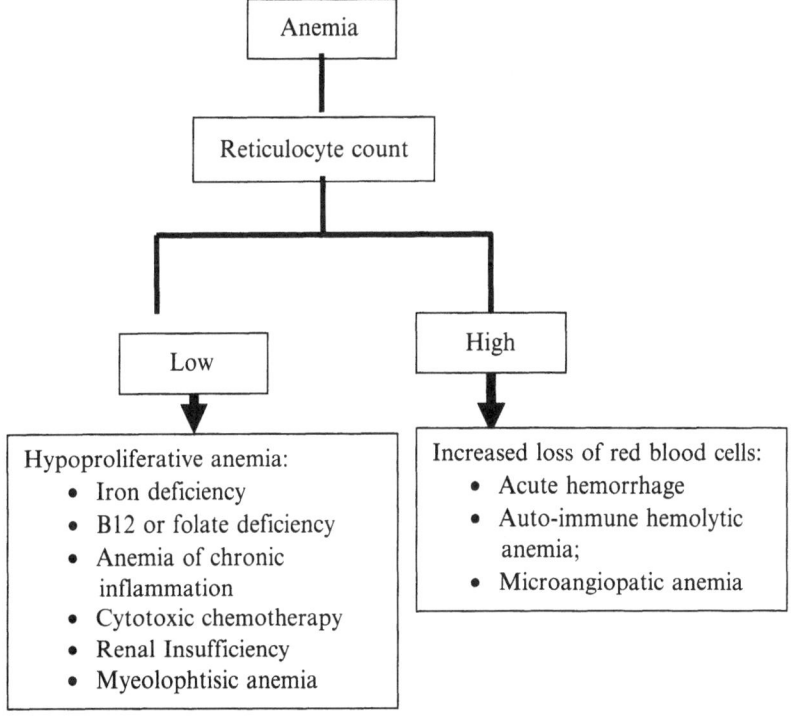

Fig. 2.4. Anemia work-up

An examination of the bone marrow should be performed when there is pancytopenia, suggesting myelophtysis. Examination of the bone marrow with cytogenetics may also be necessary for the diagnosis of MDS.

Iron deficiency is characterized by low serum iron, increased serum iron capacity, low ferritine levels and high concentrations of soluble transferrin receptors, while the ACI is characterized by low serum iron and iron binding capacity, high levels of ferritine and low concentrations of soluble transferrin receptors (41). A diagnosis of iron deficiency mandates investigations of blood loss through the digestive tract. More rarely iron deficiency may be due to loss of iron in the urine from chronic intravascular hemolytic anemia, suggested by hemosiderin in the urines.

Though the lowest levels of cobalamine in the blood are listed as 180 pg/ml, about 15% of individuals with values between 180 and 300 pg/ml have increased levels of methyl malonic acid (MMA) in the circulation suggesting functional cobalamine deficiency (69).

Anemia from chronic renal insufficiency should be suspected in all individuals whose creatinine clearance is lower than 60 ml/min and can be confirmed by levels of erythropoietin inadequate for the degree of anemia (34).

Treatment of Anemia

The treatment consists in elimination of the cause (ex. gastro-intestinal bleeding) and replacement of the missing nutrient (example iron).

Older individuals may be unable to absorb oral iron due to stomach achilia and to increased concentration of hepcidine, so they may need IV replacement.

B12 deficiency may be corrected orally, as most older people can absorb crystalline B12.

Erythropoietic growth factors should be used only for anemia of renal insufficiency and for cancer-chemotherapy related anemia. In the case of anemia of aging or other forms of ACI the benefits of erythropoietin should be explored in randomized controlled study having as end-points survival, compression of morbidity, and preservation of independence.

Conclusions

Anemia becomes more common with age and is associated with decreased survival, functional dependence, coronary deaths, congestive heart failure, and a number of geriatric syndromes, including dementia delirium, depression and falls.

In approximately one third of cases, the cause of anemia was not apparent. A number of these cases may be due to early myelodysplasia or undetected kidney insufficiency. A number of cases may be due to relative erythropoietin insufficiency, due to the pro-inflammatory status of aging.

Investigations of anemia should be initiated for hemoglobin levels lower than 13 both in man and women. In some individuals, especially women and African-Americans levels of hemoglobin between 12 and 13 gm/dl should be considered normal, if no cause of anemia is detected and the hemoglobin levels do not change for one year or longer.

The management of anemia consists in eliminating its causes and replenishing the missing factors. Currently there is no proof that management of anemia of aging with erythopoietic growth factors is beneficial. This issue should be tested in randomized controlled trials.

References

1. US life tables
2. Pitsenberger DH: Juggling work and elder caregiving: work-life balance for aging American workers. AAOHN J. 2006 Apr;54(4):181–5
3. Chapman DP, Williams SN, Strine TW et al: Dementia and its implications for public health. Prev Chronic Dis. 2006 Apr;3(2):A34. Epub 2006
4. Liao I, McGee DL, Cao G et al: Quality of the last year of life of older adults: 1986 vs 1993. JAMA. 2000;283:512–8
5. Fries GF: Aging, natural death, and the compression of morbidity. 1980. Bull W Health Org. 2002;80:245–50
6. Guralnik JM, Eisenstaedt RS, Ferrucci L, Klein HG, Woodman RC: Prevalence of anemia in persons 65 years and older in the United States: evidence for a high rate of unexplained anemia. Blood. 2004 Oct 15;104(8):2263–8
7. Beghe C, Wilson A, Ershler WB: Prevalence and outcomes of anemia in geriatrics: a systematic review of the literature. Am J Med. 2004 Apr 5;116 Suppl 7A:3S–10S
8. Anía BJ, Suman VJ, Fairbanks VF, Rademacher DM, Melton LJ 3rd: Incidence of anemia in older people: an epidemiologic study in a well defined population. J Am Geriatr Soc. 1997 Jul;45:825–31
9. Lipsitz LA: Physiological complexity, aging, and the path to frailty. Sci Aging Knowledge Environ. 2004 Apr 21;2004(16):pe16. Review
10. Walston A, Headley EC, Ferrucci L et al: Research agenda for frailty in older adults: toward a better understanding of physiology and etiology: summary from the American Geriatrics Society/National Institute on Aging Research Conference on Frailty in Older Adults. J Am Geriatr Soc. 2006 Jun;54(6):991–1001
11. Ferrucci L, Corsi A, Lauretani F, Bandinelli S, Bartali B, Taub DD, Guralnik JM, Longo DL: The origin of age-related proinflammatory state. Blood. 2005 A March 15;105(6):2294–9A
12. Duthie et al: In: Balducci L; Lyman GH, Ershler WB, Extermann M: Comprehensive Geriatric Oncology 2nd edition, Taylor & Francis, London, 2004
13. Ganz T: Regulation of iron metabolism. In: Balducci L, Ershler WB, DeGaetano G: Blood Disorders in the Elderly. Cambridge Academic Press, Cambridge 2006

14. Maggio, Cappola AR, Ceda GP et al: The hormonal pathway to frailty in older men. J Endocrinol Invest. 2005;28(11 Suppl Proceedings):15–9

15. Balducci L, Hardy CL, Lyman GH: Hemopoiesis and aging. Cancer Treat Res. 2005;124:109–31

16. Lee SJ, Lindquist K, Segal MR et al: Development and validation of a prognostic index for 4-year mortality in older adults. JAMA. 2006 Feb 15;295(7):801–8. Erratum in: JAMA. 2006 Apr 26;295(16):1900

17. Balducci L, Extermann M: The assessment of the older cancer patient. In: Balducci L, Lyman GH, Ershler WB, Extermann M: Comprehensive Geriatric Oncology 2nd edition, Taylor and Francis, London, 2004

18. Extermann M, Overcash J, Lyman GH et al: Comorbidity and functional status are independent in older cancer patients J Clin Oncol. 1998;16:1582–7

19. Anerbo S, Wahlund LO, Lokk J: The significance of thyroid-stimulating hormone and homocysteine in the development of Alzheimer's disease in mild cognitive impairment: a 6-year follow-up study. Am J Alzheimers Dis Other Demen. 2006 Jun–Jul;21(3):182–8

20. Clarfield AM: The decreasing prevalence of reversible dementias: an updated meta-analysis. Arch Intern Med. 2003 Oct 13;163(18):2219–29

21. Lyness JM, Ling DA, Cox C et al: The importance of subsyndromal depression in older primary care patients. Prevalence and associated functional disability. J Am Ger Soc. 1999;47:647–52

22. Shaininan VB, Kuo YF, Freeman: Risk of fracture after androgen deprivation for prostate cancer. N Engl J Med. 2005;352:154–64

23. Verdery RB: Failure to thrive in old age: follow-up on a workshop. J Gerontol Biol Scie Med.1997;52:M333–6

24. Fried LP, Tangen CM, Walston J et al: Frailty in older adults: evidence for a phenotype. J Gerontol Med Sci. 2001;56A:M146–56

25. Cohen HJ, Harris T, Pieper CF: Coagulation and activation of inflammatory pathways in the development of functional decline and mortality in the elderly. Am J Med. 2003;114:180–7

26. Rockwood K, Mitnitski A, Song X et al: Long-term risks of death and institutionalization of elderly people in relation to deficit accumulation at age 70. J Am Geriatr Soc. 2006 Jun;54(6):975–9

27. Mitnitski A, Song X, Skoog I et al: Relative fitness and frailty of elderly men and women in developed countries and their relationship with mortality. J Am Geriatr Soc. 2005 Dec;53(12):2184–9

28. Ruben DB, Roth C, Kamberg D et al: Restructuring primary care practices to manage geriatric syndromes: the ACOVE-2 intervention. J Am Geriatr Soc. 2003 Dec;51(12):1787–93

29. Mitnitski A, Song X, Rockwood K: The estimation of relative fitness and frailty in community-dwelling older adults using self-report data. J Gerontol A Biol Sci Med Sci. 2004 Jun;59(6):M627–32.G

30. Chaves PH, Ashar B, Guralnik J et al: Looking at the relationship between hemoglobin concentration and prevalent mobility difficulty in older women. Should the criteria currently used to define anemia in older people be reevaluated? J Am Geriatr Soc. 2002 Jul;50(7):1257–64

31. Chaves PH, Sumba RD, Leng SX et al: Impact of anemia and cardiovascular diseases on frailty status of community dwelling women. The Women Health and Aging Studies I and II. J Gerontol A Biol Sci Med Sci. 2005;60:729–35

32. Inelmen EM, Alessio MD, Gatto MRA, et al: Descriptive analysis of the prevalence of anemia in a randomly selected sample of elderly people at home: some results of an Italian multicentric study. Aging Clin Exp Res. 1994;6:81–9

33. Yamada M, Wong FL, Suzuki G et al: Longitudinal trends of hemoglobin levels in a Japanese population-RERF's Adult Health Study Project. Eur J Haematol. 2003;70:129–35

34. Ble A, Fink J, Woodman R et al: Renal function, erythropoietin and anemia of Older Persons: The In Chianti study. Arch Intern Med. 2005;165:2222–7

35. Sipponen P, Laxen F, Huotari K et al: Prevalence of low vitamin B12 and high homocysteine in serum of an elderly male population: association with atrophic gastritis and Helicobacter Pylori Infection. Scand J Gastroenterol. 2003;38:1209–216

36. Slhub J, Jacques PF, Roenberg IH et al: Serum total homocysteine concentrations in the third National Health and nutrition Examination Survey (1991–1994): population references ranges and contribution of vitamin status to high serum concentrations. Ann Intern Med. 1999;131:331–9

37. Nemeth E, Tuttle MS, Powelson J et al: Hepcidin regulates iron efflux by binding to ferroportin and inducing its internalization. Science. 2004

38. Choi JW: Serum-soluble transferrin receptor concentrations in Helicobacter pylori-associated iron-deficiency anemia. Ann Hematol. 2006 Oct;85(10):735–7

39. Ferrucci L, Guralnik L, Woodman RC et al: Proinflammatory state and circulating erythropoietin in persons with and without anemia. Am J Med. 2005;118:1288–96B

40. Ershler WB, Sheng S, McKelvey J et al: Serum erythropoietin and aging: a longitudinal analysis. J Am Ger Soc. 2005;53:1360–65 A

41. Weiss G, Goodnough LT: Anemia of chronic disease NEJM. 2005;352:1011–23

42. Ferrucci L, Maggio M, Brandinelli S et al: Low testosterone levels and risk of anemia in older men and women. Arch Int Med. 2006;166:1380–8

43. List A, Dewald G, Bennett J et al: Lenalidomide in the myelodysplastic syndrome with chromosome 5q deletion. N Engl J Med. 2006 Oct 5;355(14):1456–65

44. Kikuchi M, Inagaki T, Shinagawa N: Five-year survival of older people with anemia: variation with hemoglobin concentration. J Am Ger Soc. 2001;49:1226–8

45. Izaks GJ, Westendorp RGJ, Knook DL: The definition of anemia in older persons. JAMA. 1999;281(18):1714–1719

46. Penninx BW, Pahor M, Woodman RC et al: Anemia in old age is associated with increased mortality and hospitalization. J Gerontol Med Sci. 2006;61:474–9

47. Zakai NA, Katz R, Hirsch C et al: A prospective study of anemia status, hemoglobin concentration, and mortality in an elderly cohort: the Cardiovascular Health Study. Arch Intern Med. 2005;165:2214–20

48. Culleton BF, Manns BJ, Zhang J et al: Impact of anemia on hospitalization and mortality in older adults. Blood. 2006 May 15;107:3841–6

49. Penninx BW, Pahor M, Cesari M et al: Anemia is associated with disability and decreased physical performance and muscle strength in the elderly. J Am Geriatr Soc. 2004;52:719–24

50. Penninx BW, Guralnik JM, Onder G et al: Anemia and decline in physical performance among older persons. Am J Med. 2003;115:104–10

51. Cesari M, Penninx BW, Lauretani F et al: Hemoglobin levels and skeletal muscle: results from the INCHIANTI study. J Gerontol A Biol Med Sci. 2004;59:238–41

52. Extermann M, Chen A, Cantor AB, Corcoran MB, Meyer J, Grendys E, Cavanaugh D, Antonek S, Camarata A, Haley WE, Balducci L: Predictors of tolerance from chemotherapy in older patients: a prospective pilot study. Eur J Cancer. 2002 Jul;38(11):1466–73

53. Schrijvers D, Highley M, DeBruyn E, Van Oosterom AT, Vermorken JB: Role of red blood cell in pharmacokinetics of chemotherapeutic agents. Anticancer Drugs 1999;10:147–53

54. Ratain MJ, Schilsky RL, Choi KE et al: Adaptive control of etoposide administration: impact of interpatient pharmacodynamic variability. Clin Pharmacol Ther. 1989;45:226–33

55. Silber JH, Fridman M, Di Paola RS et al: First-cycle blood counts and subsequent neutropenia, dose reduction or delay in early stage breast cancer therapy. J Clin Oncol. 1998;16:2392–400

56. Wolff D, Culakova E, Poniewierski MS et al: Predictors of chemotherapy-induced neutropenia and its complications: results from a prospective nationwide Registry. J Support Oncol. 2005;3(6 suppl 4):24–25

57. Joosten E, Lemiengre J, Nelis T et al: Is aneamia a risk factor for delirium in acute geriatric population? Gerontology. 2006;52:382–5

58. Maraldi C, Volpato S, Cesari M et al: Anemia, physical disability and survival in older patients with heart failure. J Card Fail. 2006;12:533–9

59. Lewis BS, Karkabi B, Jaffe R et al: Anemia and heart failure: statement of the problem. Nephrol Dial Transplant. 2005;20(suppl 7):3–6

60. Phillips S, Olimann H, Schink T et al: The impact of anaemia and kidney function in congestive heart failure and preserved systolic function. Nephrol Dial Tranplant. 2005;20:915–9

61. Elabassi W, Fraser M, Williams K et al: Prevalence and clinical complications of anemia in congestive heart failure patients followed at a specialized heart function clinic. Congest Heart Fail. 2006;12:258–64

62. Wu WC, Rathore SS, Wang Y, Radford MJ, Krumholz HM: Blood transfusions in elderly patients with acute myocardial infarction. N Engl J Med. 2001 Oct 25;345(17):1230–36

63. Pickett JL, Theberge DC, Brown WS, Schweitzer SU, Nissenson AR: Normalizing hematocrit in dialysis patients improves brain function. Am J Kidney Dis 1999;33(6):1122–30

64. Atti AR, Palmer K, Volpato S et al: Anemia increases the risk of dementia in cognitively intact elderly. Neurobiol Aging. 2006;27:278–84

65. Zamboni V, Cesari M, Zuccala G et al: Anemia and cognitive performance in hospitalized older patients: results from the GIFA study. Int J Geriatr Psychiatry. 2006;21:529–34

66. Chaves PH, Carlson MC, Ferrucci L et al: Association between mild anemia and executive function impairment in community dwelling older women: The women health and aging study II. J Am Ger Soc. 2006;54:1429–35

67. Penninx BW, Pluijm SM, Lips P et al: Late life anemia is associated with increased risk of recurrent falls. J Am Geriatr Soc. 2005;53:2106–111

68. Bohlius J, Langersiepen S, Schwarzer G et al: Recombinant human erythropoietin and overall survival in cancer patients. Results of a comprehensive meta-analysis. J Natl Cancer Inst. 2005;97:489–98

69. Norman EJ, Morrison JA: Screening elderly populations for cobalamin (vitamin B12) deficiency using the urinary methylmalonic acid assay by gas chromatography mass spectrometry. Am J Med. 1993 Jun;94(6):589–94

Chapter 3

B$_{12}$ and Iron Deficiency in the Elderly

John W. Adamson

Iron deficiency, and particularly iron deficiency as a cause of anemia, is one of the commonest nutritional deficiencies in man. According to the NHANES studies of 1999–2000, there was a 4% incidence of iron deficiency and a 2% incidence of iron deficiency anemia (IDA) in males over the age of 70 (1). In females of a comparable age, it was estimated that 7% were iron deficient and 2% actually had IDA. Iron deficiency is the most common nutritional deficiency in both developed and underdeveloped countries and, worldwide, nearly one-half billion individuals suffer from iron deficiency. [An excellent review of iron metabolism in man can be found in (2); and an in-depth overview of all aspects of iron metabolism can be found in (3).]

It is important to recognize iron deficiency since iron deficiency interferes with learning in children and cognition in adults. In the pregnant woman, iron deficiency can lead to low birth weight infants. Importantly, in the elderly, iron deficiency is frequently a sign of underlying pathology.

Laboratory Tests Used to Assess Iron Status

The laboratory tests used to assess iron status are shown in Table 3.1. The next sections examine these various tests in more detail.

Transferrin (Total Iron-Binding Capacity or TIBC)

Transferrin is the major iron transport protein in the body. Its role is to shuttle iron from storage sites and the gut to the erythroid marrow where the iron that's carried can be used for hemoglobin synthesis. Transferrin is the only major iron transporter to parenchymal cells. The amount of iron transported to non-erythroid tissues is proportional to the serum iron and, thus,

Table 3.1. Tests used to assess iron status

1. Serum iron and total iron binding capacity (TIBC; transferrin) from which the percent transferrin saturation is calculated

2. Serum ferritin

3. Soluble transferrin receptor (sTfR) protein

the percent transferrin saturation. A common misconception is that transferrin is an acute phase protein. It is a better reflection of nutritional status. However, over time, transferrin levels are related inversely to total body iron stores (4). The measurement of transferrin is a direct measurement of the protein. But from a practical point of view, the physician typically orders a TIBC, which is a functional measurement of the amount of iron that the plasma is capable of binding. The TIBC is a derived value, combining the total serum iron and the unsaturated IBC. From this, one calculates the percent transferrin saturation.

Ferritin

Ferritin is produced widely throughout the body but mostly in liver cells. Ferritin is also made by erythroid and reticuloendothelial cells and functions as an iron binding protein for storage; it is not a transport protein as is transferrin. In fact, it would perhaps be more accurate to refer to serum ferritin as serum *apo*-ferritin, since very little iron is actually bound by circulating ferritin under normal conditions.

The serum ferritin level is much maligned because ferritin is an acute phase reactant and becomes elevated with inflammation. Nevertheless, the serum ferritin is the best laboratory test available to estimate total body iron stores. The validity of this concept was established years ago when normal individuals were subjected to serial phlebotomies to create a state of iron deficiency (5). The amount of iron removed (each unit of whole blood contains approximately 220 mg of elemental iron) was then correlated with the initial plasma ferritin level. As shown in Fig. 3.1, there was a very good correlation between the amount of iron removed and the initial ferritin value.

Soluble Transferrin Receptor Protein (sTfRP)

Transferrin receptors (TfR) are found primarily on erythroid tissues and this tissue normally accounts for about 80% of the number of TfR in the body. TfR are also found on liver cells and expressed on any cell during

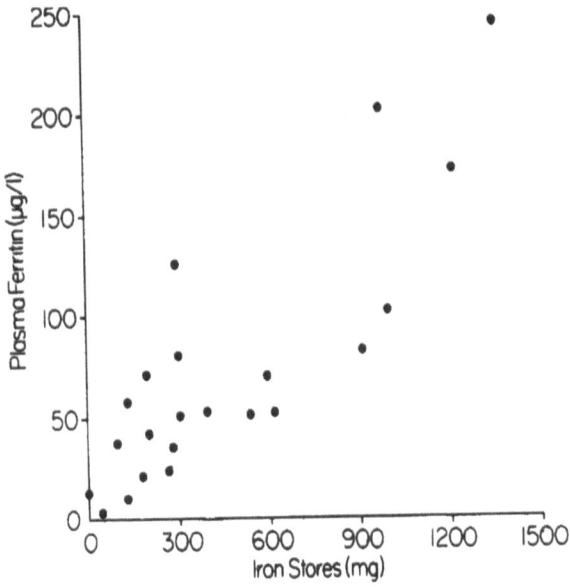

Fig. 3.1. The correlation between initial plasma ferritin concentrations and iron stores as measured by reputed venesections in a group of normal subjects (adapted from 5)

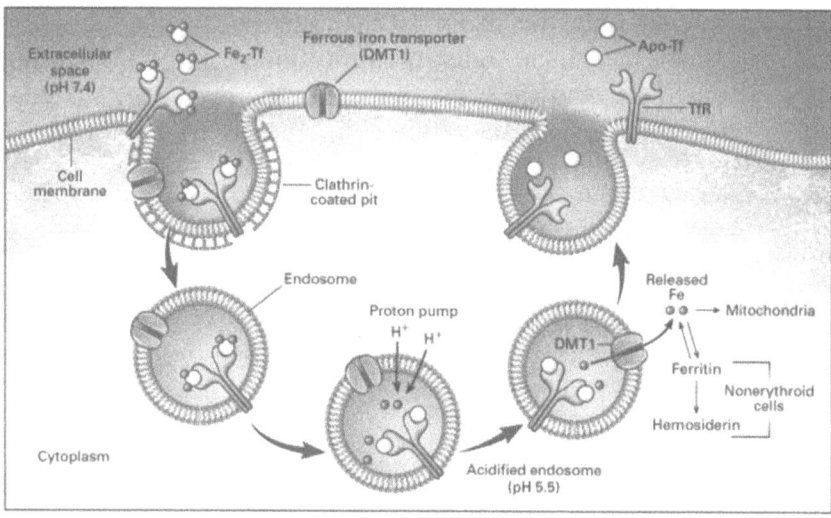

Fig. 3.2. The transferrin cycle (adapted from 2). Adapted with permission. Copyright © 1999 Massachusetts Medical Society. All rights reserved

development at a time when iron is required for growth. The TfR is recycled within developing erythroid cells, and a certain proportion is shed into the circulation as soluble TfR protein (Fig. 3.2; 2) . Thus, the amount of sTfR protein is proportional to the size of the erythroid marrow (6). However, in states of iron deficiency, the TfR gene is upregulated, and increased numbers of TfR are expressed on the surface of developing erythroid cells.

Stages in the Development of Iron Deficiency

As shown in Table 3.2, the appearance of iron deficiency requires a progressive sequence of stages before there is frank anemia. The first stage is _negative iron balance_ during which there is more iron leaving the body than is coming in. If this state persists, there is a gradual loss of iron stores and that will be reflected in a fall in the serum ferritin. Throughout this period, iron is being mobilized to support hemoglobin synthesis and there are no changes in the serum iron and the percent transferrin saturation until iron stores have been exhausted. At that point, _iron-deficient erythropoiesis_ appears, and that is manifested by the release of iron deficient (hypochromic) reticulocytes into the circulation. If iron-deficient erythropoiesis persists, the hemoglobin begins to fall (anemia) and the MCV will also begin to fall.

How Does Iron Deficiency Come About?

There are really only two major mechanisms by which iron deficiency occurs. The first is inadequate intake or absorption of iron. This may be due to an inadequate diet, but classically is seen during pregnancy, infancy, the rapid growth spurt during puberty, or in women who have increased

Table 3.2. Stages in the development of iron deficiency

1. Negative iron balance

2. Fall in iron stores (serum ferritin falls to <12–15 ng/mL)

3. Serum iron and transferrin saturation fall

4. Hypochromic reticulocytes appear in circulation

5. Hemoglobin falls

6. MCV falls

menstrual blood loss. The second major category, and partly overlapping with the first, is blood loss in excess of the individual's ability to absorb sufficient iron from the diet to keep up with ongoing losses. Table 3.3 (modified from (2)) shows a detailed list of conditions that can result in iron deficiency, either because of decreased intake or absorption or because of increased loss.

Table 3.3. Causes of iron deficiency (adapted from 2). Adapted with permission. Copyright © 1999 Massachusetts Medical Society. All rights reserved

Inadequate absorption
   Poor bioavailability
   Antacid therapy or high gastric pH
   Excess dietary bran, tannin, phytates or starch
   Competition from other metals (e.g., copper or lead)
   Loss or dysfunction of absorptive enterocytes
   Bowel resection
   Celiac disease
   Inflammatory bowel disease
   Intrinsic enterocyte defects

Increased loss
   Gastrointestinal blood loss
      Epistaxis
      Varices
      Gastritis
      Ulcer
      Tumor
      Meckel's diverticulum
      Parasitosis
      Milk-induced enteropathy of early childhood
      Vascular malformations
      Inflammatory bowel disease
      Diverticulosis
      Hemorrhoids
   Genitourinary blood loss
      Menorrhagia
      Cancer
      Chronic infection
   Pulmonary blood loss
      Pulmonary hemosiderosis
      Infection
   Other blood loss
      Trauma
      Excessive phlebotomy
      Large vascular malformations

What are the Diagnostic Criteria that Define IDA?

First, iron-deficient erythropoiesis occurs when the percent transferrin saturation falls into the range of 15–20%. However, it is important to realize that no transferrin saturation, by itself, is absolutely diagnostic of IDA. As discussed in the chapter on the anemia of chronic inflammation (ACI), there can be very rapid changes in the serum iron as a result of the effect of hepcidin to reduce iron absorption and, particularly, hepcidin's effect on blocking the release of iron from reticuloendothelial cells.

In contrast, a low serum ferritin level is absolutely diagnostic of iron deficiency (or at least absent marrow iron stores). Absent marrow iron stores are associated with serum ferritin levels of <12–15 ng/mL. Because ferritin is an acute phase reactant and will rise with inflammation, possible iron deficiency may exist with serum ferritin levels between 15 and 200 ng/mL and any ferritin level must be interpreted in the context of all of the clinical circumstances (4).

As a result, ACI and IDA share a number of overlapping features (Table 3.4). Evidence of iron-deficient erythropoiesis with a serum ferritin >200 ng/mL suggests ACI, while a serum ferritin <12–15 ng/mL is diagnostic of (at least) depleted iron stores. However, if there is doubt, one can obtain a bone marrow specimen and stain the specimen for iron.

An underutilized approach to distinguish IDA from ACI combines the serum ferritin level with the sTfR protein level. As reported by Punnonen et al. (7),

Table 3.4. The anemia of chronic disease and iron deficiency: similarities and differences

Iron deficiency anemia	ACD
Low serum iron	Low serum iron
High TIBC	Normal to low TIBC
Low % Tf saturation	Low % Tf saturation
Elevated red cell protoporphyin	Elevated red cell protoporphyrin
Red cell microcytosis	Normocytic to microcytic red cells
Low serum ferritin	Normal to elevated ferritin
Absent marrow iron stores; no sideroblasts	Marrow iron stores normal to increased; reduced sideroblasts
sTrR/log ferritin < 1	sTrR/log ferritin < 2

the serum ferritin level will be elevated in patients with ACI and depressed in patients with iron deficiency. The sTfR protein level will be elevated in iron deficiency and normal or depressed in patients with ACI. Neither of these tests, alone, distinguished patients with IDA from those with ACI or a small subset of patients who had both. However, when these investigators divided the sTfR protein value by the log of the serum ferritin, a result of <2 denoted ACI and values >2 captured patients with uncomplicated IDA or those with a combination of IDA and ACI (Fig. 3.3). However, this approach has not been validated for elderly patients who may have a chronic low level of inflammation.

Finally, if there is uncertainty, one can give a trial of iron replacement therapy. A clinical response to iron therapy (defined as an increase in hemoglobin of 1 gm/dL or more) is the ultimate definition of IDA.

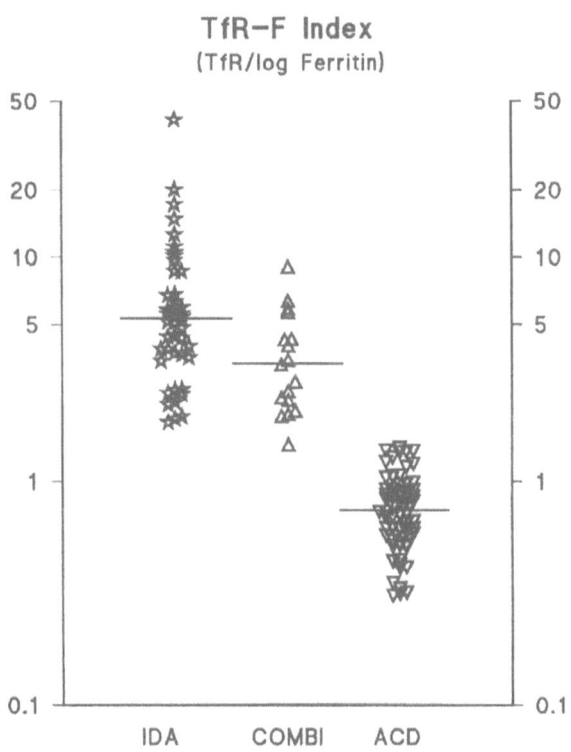

Fig. 3.3. The separation of patients with IDA, ACD or the combination of both using the sTfR/log ferritin calculation (adapted from 7). This research was originally published in *Blood.* © the American Society of Hematology

Cobalamin (Vitamin B$_{12}$) Deficiency

Vitamin B$_{12}$ (cobalamin) deficiency in the elderly is probably much more common than realized. According to the Framingham study, 12% of community dwelling elderly were cobalamin deficient (8). Other studies report as many as 30–40% of sick or institutionalized elderly are cobalamin deficient (9). In one large series from France, nearly 5% of hospitalized patients between the ages of 65 and 98 were cobalamin deficient (10).

When one looks at the mechanisms of anemia in the elderly (those 65 and above) from the NHANES study (1), iron deficiency accounted for 16.6% (and amounted to nearly one-half million individuals) while B$_{12}$ deficiency accounted for 5.9% (nearly 170,000 individuals). The combination of folic acid and B$_{12}$ deficiency added another 2% (Table 3.5).

As shown in Fig. 3.4, according to the study of Andres et al. (10), the definition of cobalamin deficiency is a serum cobalamin level <150 pmol/L on two separate occasions *or* a serum cobalamin level <150 pmol *and* a total serum homocysteine level >13 μmol/L *or* a methylmalonic acid >0.4 μmol/mL in the absence of renal failure or folate and B$_6$ deficiency. However, as pointed out by Solomon, there is considerable uncertainty about the diagnostic criteria and probably no one single laboratory value is sufficient (11). The causes of B$_{12}$ deficiency in the elderly (and the approximate frequency with which they occur) are shown in Table 3.6 (from 10).

Food cobalamin malabsorption is characterized by the inability to release cobalamin from food or from intestinal transport proteins, particularly in the presence of hypochlorhydria. This syndrome is defined by the presence of cobalamin deficiency despite an adequate diet. With this kind

---

Box 1: Definitions of cobalamin (vitamin B$_{12}$) deficiency in elderly people

- Serum cobalamin level < 150 pmol/L on 2 separate occasions

  OR

- Serum cobalamin level < 150 pmol/L AND total serum homocysteine level > 13 μmol/L OR methymalonic acid > 0.4 μmol/L (in the absence of renal failure and folate and vitamin B$_6$ deficiencies)

Fig. 3.4. Laboratory criteria for the diagnosis of B$_{12}$ deficiency in the elderly (adapted from 10)

Table 3.5. NHANES estimates of various causes of anemia in the elderly (adapted from 1). This research was originally published in *Blood*. © the American Society of Hematology

Anemia type	Number in US	Percent
Iron deficiency	467,000	16.6
Folate deficiency	181,000	6.4
B_{12} deficiency	16,600	5.9
Folate and B_{12}	56,000	2.0
Iron with others	95,000	3.4
CRF	230,000	8.2
ACI	554,000	19.7
Unexplained (UA)	945,000	33.6
Total	2,814,000	100.0

Table 3.6. Causes of B_{12} deficiency in an elderly population (adapted from 10)

1. Food cobalamin malabsorption (60–70%)

2. Pernicious anemia (15–20%)

3. Dietary deficiency (<5%)

4. Malabsorption (<5%)

5. Hereditary causes (<1%)

of malabsorption, the Schilling test, which is done with crystallized vitamin B_{12}, will be normal. The cause of food cobalamin malabsorption is predominantly due to gastric atrophy which is far more prominent in the elderly. Over 40% of patients who are over age 80 have gastric atrophy that may or may not be related to *H. pylori* infection (10). Other factors that contribute to food cobalamin malabsorption are shown in Table 3.7.

Table 3.7. Factors that contribute to malabsorption of food cobalamin (adapted from 10)

1. Intestinal microbial proliferation

2. Long-term ingestion of drugs
   Biguanides
   Antacids
   H_2 receptor antagonists
   Proton pump inhibitors

3. Chronic alcoholism

4. Gastric reconstruction

5. Pancreatic exocrine failure

6. Sjogren's syndrome

The Iron/Cobalamin Connection

H. pylori infection results in an increased gastric pH and decreased ascorbic acid secretion and eventually can lead to IDA (12, 13). It has been shown that treatment of the infection can reverse these changes and correct the iron deficiency (14).

Hershko and colleagues have explored the connection between iron deficiency and cobalamin deficiency. In a study of 150 patients with unexplained iron deficiency in Israel, these investigators noted that 27 had autoimmune gastritis as indicated by hypergastrinemia and a positive test for antiparietal cell antibodies. Of these individuals, 50% had abnormal serum cobalamin levels. Most were young women and there was a high rate of *H. pylori* infection. However, in older patients, the rate of detectable *H. pylori* infection dropped. According to the hypothesis put forward by this group, over time, the gastric mucosal niche becomes inhospitable for the bacteria, and the infection clears.

In a subsequent study, this same group stratified the patients by age and found a strong and progressive effect on all laboratory parameters. In other words, as the patients became older, there was an increased incidence of cobalamin deficiency, as shown in Table 3.8. Patients with autoimmune gastritis-associated IDA had many features overlapping with classic pernicious anemia (e.g., coincident thyroiditis, diabetes mellitus, Sjögren's syndrome, etc.). This raises the question of whether *H. pylori* gastritis represents an early phase of a progressive disease in which an infectious disease is

Table 3.8. Overlap between ID and Cbl deficiency (adapted from 15). This research was originally published in *Blood*. © the American Society of Hematology

Patient group	Cbl < 181 ng/mL	Iron deficiency
Macrocytic ($n = 29$) MCV > 100	100%	10%
Normocytic ($n = 83$)	92%	50%
Microcytic ($n = 83$) MCV < 80	46%	100%

replaced by an autoimmune disease terminating in the irreversible destruction of the gastric mucosa (13, 15).

Summary

Vitamin B_{12} deficiency in the elderly is not rare – it may not even be uncommon. Vitamin B_{12} and iron deficiencies frequently coexist and, in some patients, may have a common pathogenesis in *H. pylori* infection. Diagnostic testing may not be infallible and, again, if there is doubt, one should always treat the patient, because the consequences of not treating B_{12} deficiency may have significant and irreversible consequences for the patient.

References

1. Guralnik, JM, Eisenstaedt, RS, Ferrucci, L, et al. Prevalence of anemia in persons 65 years and older in the United States: evidence for a high rate of unexplained anemia. Blood 104:2263–2268, 2004.
2. Andrews, NC. Medical Progress: disorders of iron metabolism. N Eng J Med 341:1986–1995, 1999.
3. TH Bothwell, RW Charlton, JD Cook and CA Finch (Eds.). Iron Metabolism in Man. Blackwell Scientific Publications, Oxford, UK, 1979.
4. Lipschitz, DA, Cook, JD and Finch, CA. A clinical observation of serum ferritin. N Eng J Med 290:1213–1216, 1974.
5. Walters, GO, Miller, FM and Worwood, M. Serum ferritin concentration and iron stores in normal subjects. J Clin Path 26:770–772, 1973.
6. Huebers, HA, Beguin, Y, Pootrakul, P, et al. Intact transferrin receptors in human plasma and their relation to erythropoiesis. Blood 75:102–107, 1990.
7. Punnonen, K, Irjala, K and Rajamaki, A. Serum transferrin receptor and its ratio to serum ferritin in the diagnosis of iron deficiency. Blood 89:1052–1057, 1997.
8. Lindenbaum, J, Rosenberg, IH, Wilson, PWF, et al. Prevalence of cobalamin deficiency in the Framingham elderly population. Am J Clin Nutr 60:2–11, 1994.

9. Van Asselt, DZ, Blom, HJ, Zuiderent, R, et al. Clinical significance of low cobalamin levels in older hospital patients. Neth J Med 57:41–49, 2000.

10. Andres, E, Loukili, NH, Noel, E, et al. Vitamin B$_{12}$ (cobalamin) deficiency in elderly patients. Can Med Assoc J 171:251–259, 2004.

11. Solomon, LR. Cobalamin-responsive disorders in the ambulatory care setting: unreliability of cobalamin, methylmalonic acid, and homocysteine testing. Blood 105:978–985, 2005.

12. Annibale, B, Capurso, G, Lahner, E, et al. Concomitant alterations in intragastric pH and ascorbic acid concentration in patients with *Helicobacter pylori* gastritis and associated iron deficiency. Gut 52:496–501, 2003.

13. Hershko, C, Hoffbrand, AV, Keret, D, et al. Role of autoimmune gastritis, *Helicobacter pylori* and celiac disease in refractory unexplained iron deficiency anemia. Haematologica 90:585–595, 2005.

14. Annibale, B, Marignani, M, Monarca, B, et al. Reversal of iron deficiency anemia after *Helicobacter pylori* eradication in patients with asymptomatic gastritis. Ann Int Med 131:668–672, 1999.

15. Hershko, C, Ronson, A, Souroujon, M, et al. Variable hematologic presentation of autoimmune gastritis: age-related progression from iron deficiency to cobalamin depletion. Blood 107:1673–1679, 2006.

Chapter 4

The Anemia of Chronic Inflammation

John W. Adamson

The anemia of chronic inflammation (ACI) is one of the major causes of hypoproliferative anemia in man. ACI can be associated with inflammation of any type (Table 4.1). In each case, the associations represent a form of inflammation and cytokine release, whether infectious or not. Even with simple tissue injury, such as myocardial infarction or surgery, there is an inflammatory response in the process of wound repair.

There are four major mechanisms that contribute to the anemia of chronic inflammation.

Impaired Erythropoietin (Epo) Production

As shown by a number of investigators, patients with a variety of inflammatory conditions, including cancer or connective tissue disorders, have a blunted Epo response for the degree of anemia that is present (1). Thus, the typical logarithmic increase in plasma or urine Epo levels seen with increasing anemia is lost in patients with ACI (2).

An elegant series of experiments was carried out by Faquin et al. (3). They established cultures of the human hepatoma cell line, Hep3b. These cells have the useful property of upregulating Epo gene expression in response to hypoxia and secreting Epo into the medium (4). The results demonstrated that when inflammatory cytokines such as Interleukin-1 (IL-1) or tumor necrosis factor α (TNFα) were added to the cultures, Epo production in response to hypoxia was dramatically reduced (Fig. 4.1). The suppressive effect of the cytokines was dose-dependent and these investigators established a hierarchy of effects with IL-1β being more suppressive than IL-1α which, in turn, was followed by TNFα and TGFβ. Not only was Epo messenger RNA reduced in the presence of the inflammatory cytokines, but the amount of immunoreactive Epo secreted into the culture medium was similarly reduced.

Table 4.1. Conditions Associated with ACI

1. Acute and chronic infection (viral, bacterial, protozoal)

2. Autoimmune disease (e.g., rheumatoid arthritis)

3. Tissue injury (e.g., surgery, trauma, myocardial infarction, menses)

4. Neoplasms

5. Chronic renal failure

6. Aging

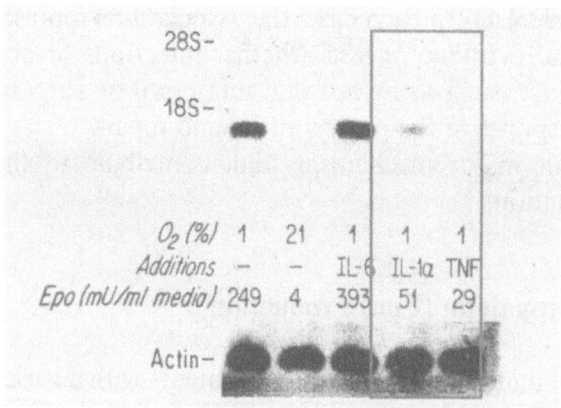

Fig. 4.1. Effect of IL-1 and TNF on erythropoietin gene expression (adapted from 3). This research was originally published in *Blood.* © the American Society of Hematology

Impaired Response of Erythroid Progenitor Cells to Epo

Cultures of erythroid colony-forming cells (CFU-E) were used to determine the effect of the same inflammatory cytokines on the progenitor cell response to Epo. Means et al. showed that many of the same inflammatory cytokines previously shown to blunt Epo production in response to hypoxia also impaired progenitor growth in the presence of Epo (5–8). Again, hierarchies based on dose and the inflammatory cytokine employed could be established. In important experiments, increasing concentrations of Epo were added to the cultures in the presence of a fixed amount of inflammatory cytokine. For many of the cytokines, the addition of greater than physiologic concentrations of Epo was able to overcome the suppressive effect of the cytokine. This set the stage for understanding the different Epo dose requirements to correct the anemia in some patient groups, such as those with the anemia associated with cancer chemotherapy (9, 10).

In vivo, the administration of IL-1 had a similar effect. When a single dose of IL-1 was given to normal mice, there was a nearly 60% reduction in the number of CFU-E in the femur and spleen of the animals (11). More primitive erythroid progenitors, such as the erythroid burst forming cell (BFU-E), were unaffected. This is entirely consistent with the fact that the terminal events in erythroid progenitor cell differentiation and maturation are under the control of Epo, while the earlier events are regulated or affected by other cytokines, such as KIT-ligand or IL-3. Importantly, the suppressive effects of IL-1 on erythropoiesis in vivo could be completely reversed and, in fact, overcome by the simultaneous administration of Epo to the animals.

These studies established several important principles about Epo and ACI. First, inflammatory cytokines, which are increased in certain clinical conditions, had a direct suppressive effect on Epo production. Second, in vivo, recombinant Epo could overcome the effect of the inflammatory cytokines, paving the way for Epo therapy of the anemia associated with a variety of conditions, including the anemia of cancer chemotherapy.

The Effect of Inflammation on Iron Homeostasis

This is an area in which there have been major recent developments in our understanding of the role of inflammation on iron homeostasis. To understand this, it is important to review the major mechanisms of iron transport in man (12, 13). Normally, humans obtain iron for hemoglobin synthesis and other important cellular functions from the diet. The daily amount required is 1–2 mg of elemental iron per day. There are important mechanisms that control the absorption of iron at the level of the small intestine. Iron, which is to be absorbed from the gut, has to be presented in the appropriate (reduced) state, whereby it can be imported into the luminal cell through divalent metal transporter 1 (DMT1). Once inside the cell, the iron has two paths. It can be bound to ferritin and stored within the cell or it can be transported to the basolateral surface of the luminal cell where it can be released to transferrin for transport to the erythroid marrow and other tissues. The mechanism by which iron is exported from the luminal cell involves ferroportin, the membrane-imbedded iron exporter whose function is regulated by the iron regulatory peptide, hepcidin (see below). Once iron is bound to plasma transferrin, it circulates and most of it is utilized by the erythroid marrow for hemoglobin synthesis. Because approximately 20–25 mg of elemental iron are required to replace senescent red cells each day, and because the circulating transferrin pool only contains about 3 mg of elemental iron, the transferrin iron pool must turn over 6–8 times a day in order to provide enough iron to sustain normal hemoglobin synthesis and maintain a normal hematocrit and hemoglobin. Since only 1–2 mg/day comes in via absorption, efficient reutilization of iron harvested from senescent red cells is critical to the process. The iron from senescent red cells must be efficiently processed by reticuloendothelial (RE) cells and exported to transferrin. Thus, the flux of iron coming into the transferrin pool from the gut and from RE cells is critical for providing adequate iron for erythropoiesis. Anything that disrupts this flux will result in a fall in the serum iron and can lead to iron-deficient erythropoiesis. With inflammation, it has been recognized for many years that iron absorption decreases and the release of iron from RE storage sites is reduced. However, it has only been within the last 6 years that the actual molecular mechanism and the identification of the key iron regulatory hormone, hepcidin, have come about.

Hepcidin

Hepcidin was originally studied as an antimicrobial agent, HAMP (*hep*cidin *antimi*crobial *p*eptide). Inadvertently, investigators studying a gene important in gluconeogenesis, silenced the gene for hepcidin in a transgenic mouse experiment (14). Quite unexpectedly, the knockout mice developed hepatic and pancreatic iron overload with an absence of iron in the spleen. (Figs. 4.2 and 4.3). The pathology had all of the features of a patient with idiopathic hemochromatosis (genetically determined iron overload). In subsequent experiments, the investigators went on to overexpress the hepcidin gene in other transgenic animals (15). This resulted in mice that were severely iron deficient at birth, demonstrating the importance of hepcidin even in transplacental transport of iron to the developing fetus. The mice were born with severe microcytic hypochromic anemia and died shortly after birth, presumably because of an inability to absorb iron from the gut.

Very recently, Nemeth and coworkers defined the mechanism of action of hepcidin (16). First, cell systems were established that expressed ferroportin, the molecule critical for the export of iron from cells. Ferroportin was linked to green fluorescent protein and then the appearance of ferroportin was examined microscopically on the surface of expressing cells, both in the presence and absence of hepcidin. In the absence of hepcidin, ferroportin localized to the cell surface. The addition

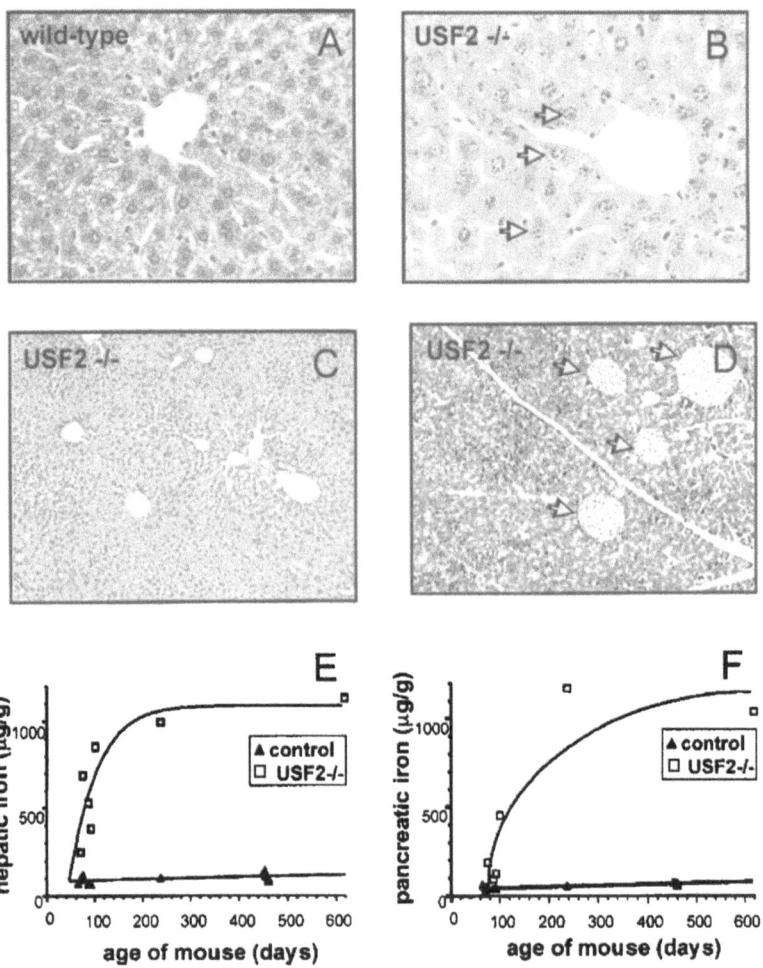

Fig. 4.2. USF2-/- mice develop hepatic and pancreatic iron overload (adapted from 14). Copyright 2001 National Academy of Sciences, U.S.A

of hepcidin to the cultures led to the internalization and lysosomal degradation of the complex. Thus, ferroportin was shown to be the receptor for hepcidin. Ferroportin is expressed predominantly on cells of the RE system as well as the abluminal cell membrane of the absorptive cells in the gut. Ferroportin is also expressed, but at lower levels, on hepatocytes. Thus, hepcidin, which is upregulated in typical conditions of iron overload, interacts with both storage cells and with absorptive cells to reduce the amount of iron available for transferrin binding.

In studies of hepcidin gene regulation, it was found that hepcidin was upregulated in patients with transfusional iron overload, as well as in patients with ACI (17). Hepcidin levels were normal in patients with hereditary

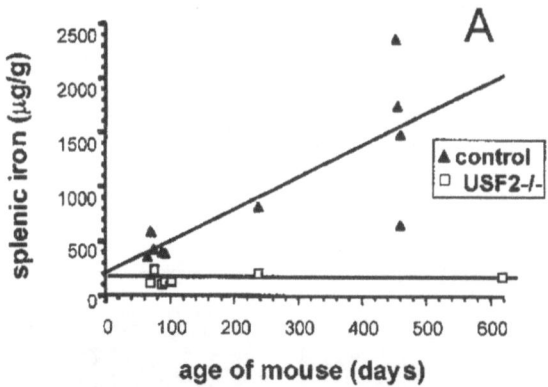

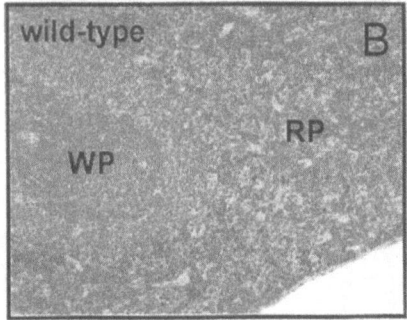
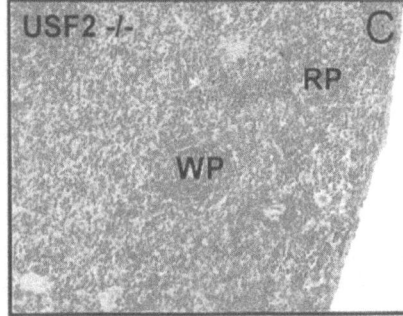

Fig. 4.3. USF2-/- mice fail to store iron in the spleen compared to wt mice (adapted from 14). Copyright 2001 National Academy of Sciences, U.S.A

hemochromatosis whose disease was controlled through phlebotomy as well as patients with iron deficiency. The molecules that specifically were involved in upregulating hepcidin expression included IL-6 and lipopolysaccharide (17, 18). Thus, hepcidin is part of the Type II inflammatory response pathway that also includes fibrinogen, haptoglobin and α1-antitrypsin. Hepcidin gene expression was down-regulated by TNFα and iron deficiency. Both in iron deficiency and iron overload, the molecular mechanisms that result in alterations in hepcidin gene expression are not fully worked out.

IL-6 turns out to be an interesting link between ACI and the anemia of aging. Ferucci (19) has shown that with aging there is a progressive increase in the average levels of cytokines, particularly IL-6, in both men and women, and that this is paralleled by increases in C-reactive protein and fibrinogen (Fig. 4.4). Consequently, some of the anemia of aging may be related to inflammation with its attendant effects on Epo production, progenitor responsiveness to Epo, and alterations in iron metabolism.

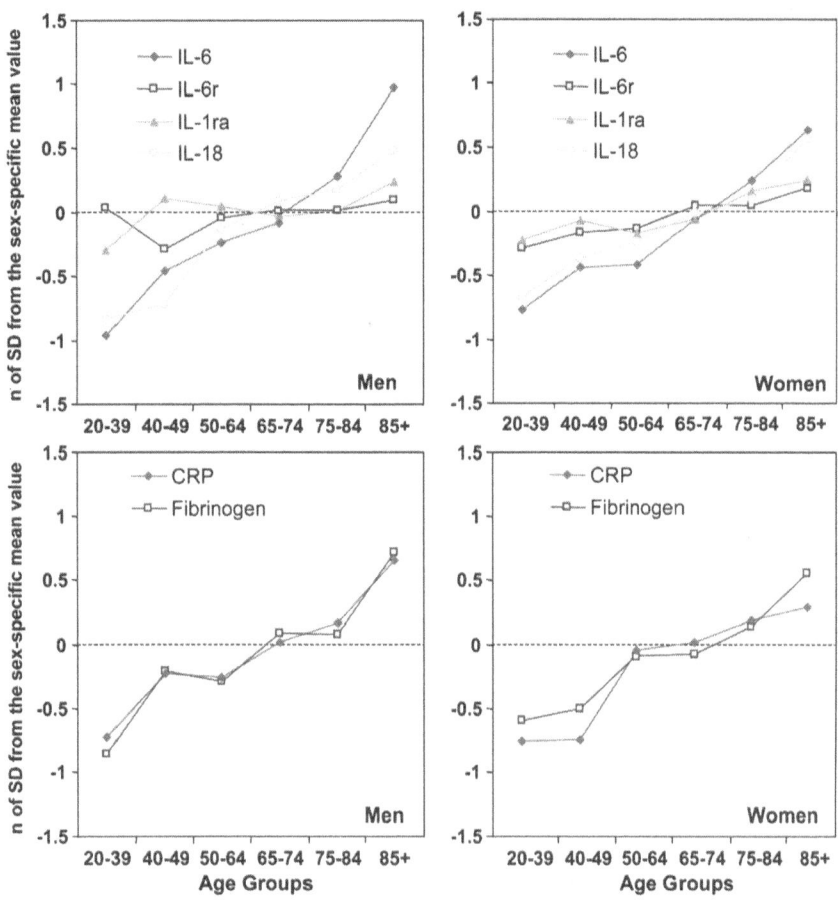

Fig. 4.4. Mean values of inflammatory markers with age (adapted from 19). This research was originally published in *Blood.* © the American Society of Hematology

In clinical studies, urinary hepcidin excretion correlates very closely with plasma ferritin levels (17). In a longitudinal clinical study of a patient with bacterial epididymitis, high hepcidin levels fell over time as the infection was adequately treated with antibiotics.

To directly demonstrate its effect on serum iron levels, hepcidin was administered to normal mice (20). Hepcidin caused a dose-dependent fall in the serum iron. In timed studies, a single injection of hepcidin resulted in a prompt fall in the serum iron which was then sustained over a period of nearly 48 h (Fig. 4.5). Thus, hepcidin becomes the central regulator of alterations in iron homeostasis in patients with ACI. Hepcidin's role may actually be broader in that at least one recent report suggests that hepcidin, itself, suppresses erythroid progenitor cell responses to Epo (21). This interesting observation remains to be confirmed.

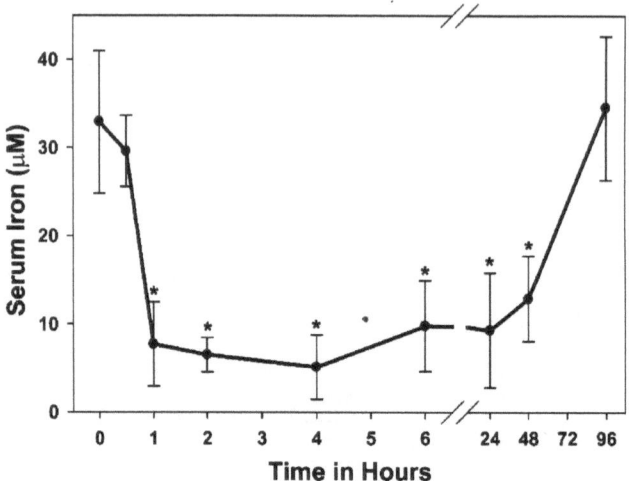

Fig. 4.5. Hepcidin causes a rapid, sustained fall in serum iron (adapted from 20). This research was originally published in *Blood*. © the American Society of Hematology

In addition to alterations in the Epo-progenitor cell axis, and alterations in iron homeostasis, ACI is also associated with a modest shortening of red cell survival (22–24). It is not certain what the mechanisms are behind the shortened survival but it may have to do with activated macrophages in the inflammatory state and enhanced recognition of effete red cells.

Summary

ACI is a multifactorial anemia with major alterations in Epo production, the response of progenitor cells to Epo, and in iron homeostasis. The key regulator of changes in iron homeostasis is hepcidin. Thus, inflammation of a variety of kinds, which accumulates over time with aging, may result in the modest hypoproliferative anemia which is so commonly seen in the elderly. At least part of the mechanisms may be mediated by IL-6 and hepcidin. This is obviously a fertile area for future investigation.

[For a recent review of the ACI, please refer to Weiss and Goodnough, ref. 25]

References

1. Miller, CB, Jones, RJ, Piantadosi, S, et al. Decreased erythropoietin response in patients with the anemia of cancer. N Eng J Med 322:1689–1692, 1990.
2. Cotes, PM and Spivak, JL. Erythropoietin and health and disease. In: Erythropoietin. Molecular, Cellular and Clinical Biology. Ed. Erslev, AJ et al. pp: 184–207, 1991. Johns Hopkins Press.

3. Faquin, WC, Schneider, TJ and Goldberg, MA. Effect of inflammatory cytokines on hypoxia-induced erythropoietin production. Blood 79:1987–1994, 1992.
4. Goldberg, MA, Glass, GA, Cunningham, JM and Bunn, HF. The regulated expression of erythropoietin by two human hepatoma cell lines. Proc Natl Acad Sci 84:7972–7976, 1987.
5. Means, RT, Dessypris, EN and Krantz, SB. Inhibition of human colony-forming units erythroid by tumor necrosis factor requires accessory cells. J Clin Invest 86:538–541, 1990.
6. Means, RT, Dessypris, EN and Krantz, SB. Inhibition of erythroid colony-forming units by interleukin-1 is mediated by gamma interferon. J Cell Physiol 150:59–64, 1992.
7. Means, RT and Krantz, SB. Inhibition of human erythroid colony-forming units by tumor necrosis factor requires beta interferon. J Clin Invest 91:416–419, 1993.
8. Means, RT, Krantz, SB, Luna J, et al. Inhibition of murine erythroid colony formation in vitro by gamma interferon and correction by interferon inhibitor. Blood 83:911–915, 1994.
9. Abels, RI. Use of recombinant human erythropoietin in the treatment of anemia in patients who have cancer. Semin Oncol 19:29–35, 1992.
10. Henry, DH and Abels, RI. Recombinant human erythropoietin in the treatment of cancer and chemotherapy-induced anemia: results of double-blind and open-label follow-up studies. Semin Oncol 21:21–28, 1994.
11. Johnson, CS, Keckler, DJ, Topper, MI, et al. In vivo hematopoietic effects of recombinant interleukin-1α in mice: stimulation of granulocytic, monocytic, megakaryocytic, and early erythroid progenitors, suppression of late-stage erythropoiesis, and reversal of erythroid suppression with erythropoietin. Blood 73:678–683, 1989.
12. Andrews, NC. Medical progress: disorders of iron metabolism. N Eng J Med 341:1986–1995, 1999.
13. Fleming, RE and Bacon, BR. Orchestration of iron homeostasis. N Eng J Med 352:1741–1744, 2005.
14. Nicolas, G, Bennoun, M, Devaux, I, et al. Lack of hepcidin gene expression and severe tissue iron overload in upstream stimulatory factor 2 (*USF2*) knockout mice. Proc Natl Acad Sci 98:8780–8785, 2001.
15. Nicolas, G, Bennoun, M, Porteu, A, et al. Severe iron deficiency anemia in transgenic mice expressing liver hepcidin. Proc Natl Acad Sci 99:4596–4601, 2002.
16. Nemeth, E, Tuttle, MS, Powelson, J, et al. Hepcidin regulates cellular iron efflux by binding to ferroportin and inducing its internalization. Science 306:2090–2093, 2004.
17. Nemeth, E, Valore, EV, Territo, M, et al. Hepcidin, a putative mediator of anemia of inflammation, is a type II acute-phase protein. Blood 101:2461–2463, 2003.
18. Nemeth, E, Rivera, S, Gabayan, V, et al. IL-6 mediates hypoferremia of inflammation by inducing the synthesis of the iron regulatory hormone, hepcidin. J Clin Invest 113:1271–1276, 2004.
19. Ferrucci, L, Corsi, A, Lauretani, F, et al. The origins of age-related proinflammatory state. Blood 105:2294–2299, 2005.
20. Rivera, S, Nemeth, E, Gabayan, V, et al. Synthetic hepcidin causes rapid dose-dependent hypoferremia and is concentrated in ferroportin-containing organs. Blood 106:2196–2199, 2005.
21. Dallalio, G, Law, E and Means, RT. Hepcin inhibits in vitro erythroid colony formation at reduced erythropoietin concentrations. Blood 107:2702–2704, 2006.
22. Cartwright, GE. The anemia of chronic disorders. Semin Hematol 3:351–375, 1966.
23. Lee, GR. The anemia of chronic disease. Semin Hematol 20:61–79, 1983.
24. Moldawer, LL, Marano, MA, Wei, H, et al. Cachectin/tumor necrosis factor-α alters red blood cell kinetics and induces anemia in vivo. FASEB J 3:1637–1643, 1989.
25. Weiss, G and Goodnough, LT. Anemia of chronic disease. N Eng J Med 352:1011–1023, 2005.

Chapter 5

Anemia due to Chronic Kidney Disease in the Elderly

Jeffrey S. Berns

Introduction

Anemia is a well-known complication of chronic kidney disease (CKD) that develops as kidney function declines. In most patients with CKD, the glomerular filtration rate (GFR) declines over time, and as it does so, anemia becomes more prevalent and more severe. The relationship between anemia and CKD in elderly subjects is not as well defined as in younger populations. As discussed elsewhere in this book, the optimal definition of anemia in older subjects is a matter of some debate (1, 2). Also, the estimation of the level of kidney function in older individuals poses some special problems that will be discussed.

Since the association of anemia and reduced kidney function in the general (i.e., non-elderly) population is discussed thoroughly elsewhere (3–5), this chapter focuses on specific issues pertinent to the assessment of kidney function in the elderly, the diagnosis and impact of CKD-related anemia in the elderly, and treatment of anemia in elderly subjects with CKD-related anemia.

Assessment of Kidney Function in the Elderly

Kidney function commonly declines with age, although not universally (6–9). Approximately one-third of elderly adults do not exhibit an age-related decline in kidney function (6). This has led to the suggestion that a decline in GFR is not a normal accompaniment of aging, but rather due at least in part to concomitant hypertension, cardiovascular disease, and diabetes mellitus. By the age of 80 years, mean GFR, depending on how it is measured or estimated, is approximately 50–80 mL/min, compared to

120 mL/min or greater in subjects in their 20s–40s. The prevalence of CKD in 65–74 year olds and individuals 75 years and greater is increasingly steadily, and there are more patients 70 years or older starting dialysis each year than any other age group (10). Despite this reduced level of GFR with advanced age, serum creatinine levels tend to remain relatively unchanged or increase only modestly over time in the absence of other conditions, a reflection of the reduced muscle mass that often accompanies aging (6, 11, 12).

Until recently, in routine clinical practice kidney function has been most commonly assessed by simple measurement of serum creatinine, collection of a 24-h urine for creatinine clearance, or use of simple equations, such as the Cockcroft–Gault equation (Table 5.1), to estimate GFR. In the elderly, reduction in muscle mass compared to younger subjects distorts the relationship between serum creatinine and estimated GFR (eGFR) using the Cockcroft–Gault formula so that serum creatinine typically underestimates the severity of CKD. Further complicating discussion of impaired kidney function has been the use of undefined terms such as "chronic renal failure" and "chronic renal insufficiency."

Recent developments have greatly improved the clinical evaluation of kidney function. First, as the result of the analysis of a wealth of data from the Modification of Diet in Renal Disease (MDRD) Study, prediction equations were derived that can more precisely provide an eGFR than previously available methods, including 24-h urine collections (13). While still imperfect due to lack of a standardized serum creatinine assay (a national standard is expected in the US in 2008) and uncertain validity in certain populations (such as the elderly; see below), use of the so-called abbreviated or modified MDRD prediction equation (Table 5.1) has increasingly gained acceptance as an important clinical tool for assessing

Table 5.1. Cockcroft–Gault and abbreviated MDRD prediction equations

---

Cockcroft-Gault formula:

$$\text{Creatinine clearance (ml/min)} = \frac{(140-\text{age}) \times (\text{weight})}{72 \times S_{cr}} \ (\times \, 0.85 \text{ if female})$$

Abbreviated (4-variable) MDRD equation:

$$\text{Estimated GFR (mL/min/1.73 m}^2) = 186 \times (S_{cr})^{-1.154} \times (\text{age})^{-0.203} \times (0.742 \text{ if female}) \times (1.210 \text{ if black})$$

S_{cr} = serum creatinine; age in years; weight in kg

Table 5.2. Stages of chronic kidney disease

Stage	Description	GFR (mL/min/1.73 m^2)
1	Kidney damage with normal or increased GFR	≥90
2	Kidney damage with mild decrease in GFR	60–89
3	Moderate decrease in GFR	30–59
4	Severe decrease in GFR	15–29
5	Kidney failure	<15 (or dialysis)

Chronic kidney disease is defined as a GFR < 60 mL/min/1.73 m^2 for 3 or more months, or the presence of structural or functional abnormalities of the kidneys (pathologic abnormalities or abnormal findings on blood or urine tests or in imaging studies), with or without decreased GFR, for at least 3 months.
Adapted from (14).

GFR. More recently, the National Kidney Foundation's Kidney Disease Outcomes Quality Initiative (KDOQI) Chronic Kidney Disease Workgroup published a CKD classification scheme that has quickly been adopted by the renal community (Table 5.2) (14). Thus, in 2007 we find ourselves with improved prediction equations for determination of eGFR and a useful schema for categorizing levels of CKD.

The Cockcroft–Gault formula was derived over 30 years ago from 236 hospitalized men between the ages of 18 and 92 years (15). Several MDRD equations, with the 4-variable version in most common use, were derived and validated in 1,628 subjects (mean age of 50.6 years) with precise GFR measurements and laboratory data (13), thus their generalizability to older subjects was initially unclear. A few studies have recently evaluated the Cockcroft–Gault and MDRD equations in the elderly.

Fehrman-Ekholm and Skeppholm (8) measured kidney function with the iohexol clearance method as the gold standard against which other formulae were compared in 52 Swedish subjects between the ages of 71 and 110 years (mean 82.3 years). The mean iohexol GFR was 67.7 mL/min/1.73 m^2. One of the MDRD equations (using serum creatinine, age, gender, age, BUN, and serum albumin) and the Cockcroft–Gault formula both correlated reasonably well (R^2 = 0.53 and 0.50, respectively), although the Cockcroft–Gault formula tended to systematically underestimate GFR. Verhave and colleagues (16) compared the Cockcroft–Gault formula and modified MDRD equation (using serum creatinine, gender, and age) with ^{99m}Tc-DTPA renal clearance measurements in 850 subjects as old as 93 years. Among subjects 65 years or older, both the Cockcroft–Gault formula

Table 5.3. Serum creatinine concentrations corresponding to eGFR levels of 60 mL/min/1.73 m² by the abbreviated MDRD equation or 60 mL/min by the Cockcroft–Gault equation

| Age (Yrs) | MDRD Equation | | | | Cockcroft–Gault formula | |
| | European-American | | African-American | | | |
	Men	Women	Men	Women	Men	Women
50	1.34	1.03	1.58	1.22	1.50	1.28
60	1.30	1.00	1.53	1.18	1.33	1.13
70	1.26	0.97	1.49	1.15	1.17	0.99
80	1.23	0.95	1.46	1.12	1.00	0.85

Calculations assume weight of 72 kg and body surface area of 1.73 m². Creatinine in mg/dL. Adapted from (14).

and MDRD formula both underestimated GFR, with the magnitude of the underestimate influenced by the creatinine assay methodology. The Cockcroft–Gault formula underestimated mean GFR by 11.3–20.2 mL/min/1.73 m² and the MDRD formula underestimated mean GFR by 3.7–17.8 mL/min/1.73 m². Other investigators have also reported a greater degree of underestimation of GFR in elderly patients using the Cockcroft–Gault formula compared to the MDRD equations (17, 18). This tendency for greater underestimation of GFR with the Cockcroft–Gault formula leads to the inevitable conclusion that the prevalence of CKD is substantially lower if one uses the MDRD equations rather than Cockcroft–Gault formula, regardless of which is more accurate (19).

The need to avoid dependence on serum creatinine levels, particularly in the elderly, is made apparent in Table 5.3, showing the level of serum creatinine above which eGFR is below 60 mL/min/1.73 m² or estimated creatinine clearance is below 60 mL/min, i.e., stage 3 CKD or less. Other methods for assessing kidney function, such as use of plasma cystatin C concentration, remain to be validated in the elderly, and are not yet in generally widespread use (20–22).

Anemia due to CKD in the Elderly

A normochromic normocytic anemia is a well-known complication of CKD (4, 5). Recent findings from the NHANES III study (in which the mean age was 48 years) indicate that Hgb levels typically begin to decline as the GFR falls below 70 mL/min in men and 50 mL/min in women, and that the prevalence and severity of anemia increase as kidney function falls below a level of about 60 mL/min. The prevalence of Hgb levels below 11 g/dL increases as GFR falls below about 30 mL/min/1.73 m^2 (5, 14, 23–25). The principal underlying etiology of CKD-related anemia is impaired synthesis of the glycoprotein hormone erythropoietin, which is produced primarily in peritubular cells of the kidneys. Other important contributing factors include the presence of inhibitors of erythropoiesis, reduced red cell lifespan, iron deficiency, vitamin B12 and folate deficiency, blood loss due to phlebotomy and surgery, other underlying disease processes such as infection, inflammation, poor nutritional status, hemolysis, multiple myeloma, malignancy, HIV infection, and among dialysis patients, dialysis-related blood losses and severe hyperparathyroidism. Many of these conditions are likely to be more prevalent in the elderly than in younger subjects (26).

CKD has been reported to be the principal cause of anemia in more than 8% of older subjects, and a contributing cause in others (27). The pathophysiologic basis for anemia related to CKD in older individuals is likely similar to that of younger subjects, complicated perhaps by a greater impact of underlying inflammatory processes, and in men, an age-related decline in testosterone levels (28). Although information is conflicting, data from the Baltimore Longitudinal Study on Aging revealed a rise in serum erythropoietin level over time in that sample of older adults, regardless of the presence or absence of anemia (29, 30). The increase in erythropoietin levels was less marked in subjects with hypertension or diabetes mellitus, perhaps reflecting some underlying CKD, either age-related or due to these other conditions. While some studies suggest that the erythropoietin production in response to anemia and erythropoietin responsiveness is blunted in healthy elderly subjects, others have found no difference comparing older and younger subjects, and most have not considered the effect of underlying CKD (25, 29–36).

One assessment of the association of anemia and CKD in the elderly comes from the InCHIANTI study, a prospective, population-based survey of older residents of Tuscany, Italy, who were 65 years older (mean 74.5 years; range 65–102 years) and in whom anemia was defined using the WHO criteria (Hgb < 12 g/dL in women and <13 g/dL in men) (37). Kidney function was measured with 24-h urine collections for creatinine clearance. In both men and women, the prevalence of anemia was greater at older ages, and both Hgb and creatinine clearance declined with increasing age. The mean age-related decline in Hgb and creatinine clearance was 0.75 g/dL and 19.4 mL/min per decade, respectively, in men, and 0.50 g/dL and 15.2 mL/min per decade, respectively, in women. The unadjusted prevalence of anemia, using WHO criteria, was higher among men and women at lower levels of creatinine clearance, particularly among subjects with creatinine clearance of 60 mL/min or less; 6.6% in subjects with creatinine clearance greater than 90%, 9.8% in those with creatinine clearance of 61–90 mL/min, 18.5% among those with creatinine clearance of 31–60 mL/min, and 65.4% in those with creatinine clearance of 30 mL/min or less. In age- and sex-adjusted comparisons, the prevalence of anemia was greater only in the group with creatinine clearance levels of 30 mL/min or less. Serum erythropoietin levels declined with lower levels of kidney function, although age- and Hgb-adjusted levels were significantly lower, compared to the group with creatinine clearance greater than 90 mL/min, only in subjects with creatinine clearance of 30 mL/min or less. The authors of this study concluded that among older individuals, the age-related decline in erythropoietin synthesis was an important contributing factor to anemia only when kidney function was severely impaired, i.e., when creatinine clearance was 30 mL/min or less.

In an earlier study of subjects between the ages of 49 and 97 years, there was also an inverse relationship between creatinine clearance (estimated with the Cockcroft–Gault formula) and prevalence of anemia (using WHO criteria), with a greater than fivefold risk of anemia among men and greater than threefold risk of anemia in women with creatinine clearance less than 50 mL/min compared to those with higher creatinine clearance (12). It was estimated that approximately 82% of cases of anemia in women and 68% of cases of anemia in men with CKD could be attributed to their CKD. In the entire study population, it was estimated that in approximately 17% of women and 22% of men, anemia could be attributed to renal impairment.

Effects of Anemia on Elderly Patients with CKD

In the general population with CKD, anemia has clearly been associated with reduced mortality and quality of life (QOL), increased hospitalization risk and longer hospital stays, reduced exercise capacity, and greater cardiovascular and cerebrovascular disease burden. Less is known of the anemia-related impact specifically among elderly subjects with CKD. This was assessed in a recent prospective study of more than 17,000 residents of Calgary, Canada who were 66 years of age or older (38). Anemia was associated with a fivefold increase in the risk for all-cause mortality in an adjusted analysis. When assessed in terms of baseline GFR, the hazard ratio for mortality risk associated with anemia in subjects with a normal GFR was 4.29, compared to 2.80 in subjects with a GFR of 30–59 mL/min/1.73 m^2, and 1.53 in those with a GFR less than 30 mL/min/1.73 m^2.

Thus, the incremental risk associated with anemia was actually greater at higher levels of kidney function than at lower levels, although in both anemic and nonanemic subjects, lower levels of GFR were associated with higher mortality.

In a retrospective study of patients aged 67 years or older using a Medicare database 5% sample, anemia was associated with increased risk of atherosclerotic vascular disease, congestive heart failure, renal replacement therapy, and death (39). Anemia may also be a risk factor for cognitive impairment associated with CKD in the elderly (40).

Among nonelderly subjects with CKD, anemia has been associated with substantially increased medical, as well as nonmedical (i.e., indirect costs such as sick leave, disability, etc.) costs (41, 42). Using analysis of approximately 6 years of medical and pharmacy claims from a large managed care database, Lefebvre and colleagues (43) assessed costs associated with untreated anemia in 2001 subjects 65 years of age or older with eGFR less than 60 mL/min/1.73 m^2. Observation periods with and without anemia were compared. Untreated anemia was associated with a significant increase in health care costs; compared to periods of time when anemia was not present, monthly costs for outpatient services, inpatient services, and total costs were 1.4 to 2-fold higher. Inpatient services were the most significant factor associated with higher costs in anemic compared to nonanemic periods. Pharmacy costs were not higher during periods of untreated anemia. In multivariate analysis, it was determined that the cost burden of anemia in these older subjects was comparable to those associated with diabetes, coronary artery disease, and other comorbidities. The lower the Hgb level and GFR, the higher the overall costs of care.

Treatment of Anemia in Elderly Patients with CKD

Recombinant human erythropoietin (epoetin) therapy revolutionized the treatment of anemia in patients on dialysis with CKD not receiving dialysis (44, 45). More recently, a longer-acting darbepoetin alfa erythropoiesis stimulating agent (ESA) has become available (46–49), and soon, newer form with varying mechanisms of action will likely become available for clinical use (46, 50). The risks and benefits of epoetin and darbepoetin therapy in the general population of patients with CKD have been well recognized and will not be addressed here further. Unfortunately, the specific risks and benefits, as well costs, of such treatment in the elderly have not been well characterized.

Among normal (i.e., no CKD) elderly subjects, responsiveness to exogenous epoetin does not appear to be impaired compared to younger subjects

(32, 51). Limited data suggest that epoetin responsiveness in older dialysis patients is similar to younger patients (52, 53). Despite similar monthly epoetin doses, the mean monthly Hgb level among dialysis patients 75 years and older tend to be lower than younger patients, suggesting that this population group are not substantially hyporesponsive to epoetin therapy (10).

Among elderly hemodialysis patients, the impact of epoetin therapy on QOL has been mixed. While one small study questioned the benefit (54), a larger, controlled trial found that the improvements in QOL scores after 6 month of epoetin treatment were of similar magnitude in hemodialysis patients 60 years of age and older compared to those less than 60 years, although absolute QOL scores were lower both before and after treatment in the older subjects (55).

Given the limited data available, elderly patients with CKD, whether on dialysis or not, should probably be evaluated and treated for their anemia as generally recommended for patients with CKD regardless of age (5). The most recent clinical practice guidelines and recommendations for the National Kidney Foundation KDOQI for Anemia in CKD recommend that Hgb testing be carried out at least annually in all patients with CKD, regardless of stage or cause, and that a diagnosis of anemia should be made and evaluation should be undertaken when the Hgb level is less than 13.5 g/dL in adult males and 12.0 g/dL in adult females. This evaluation should include a complete blood count (CBC), red blood cell indices (mean corpuscular hemoglobin [MCH], mean corpuscular volume [MCV], mean corpuscular hemoglobin concentration [MCHC]), white blood cell count, and differential and platelet count, absolute reticulocyte count, serum ferritin to assess iron stores, and serum TSAT or content of Hb in reticulocytes (CHr) to assess adequacy of iron for erythropoiesis.

Among patients treated with ESA therapy and/or iron, the recommended lower limit of Hgb in patients with CKD is 11.0 g/dL. In the opinion of the KDOQI Anemia Work Group, there was insufficient evidence to recommend routinely maintaining Hgb levels at 13.0 g/dL or greater in ESA-treated patients. Since adequate iron stores are essential for optimal erythropoiesis, with or without ESA therapy, the Anemia Work Group recommended that sufficient iron should be administered to generally maintain the serum ferritin concentration greater than 200 ng/mL in hemodialysis patients and greater than 100 ng/mL in CKD patients not on dialysis and those on peritoneal dialysis, with a TSAT greater than 20% in all patients. In addition, in the opinion of the Work Group, there was insufficient evidence to recommend routine administration of IV iron if serum ferritin level is greater than 500 ng/mL. When ferritin level is greater than 500 ng/mL, decisions regarding IV iron administration need to consider ESA responsiveness, Hgb levels over time, the TSAT level, and the patient's clinical status.

Recent studies have reinforced the recommendation to maintain Hgb levels below 13 g/dL, and have raised concern that even this level of anemia correction may be excessive in patients with CKD. A randomized, controlled trial in hemodialysis patients, which compared a target hematocrit level of 30% versus 42%, was stopped early when it became apparent that there was no benefit in patients assigned to the higher hematocrit target (56). The risk of the primary composite outcome of first nonfatal myocardial infarction or death was 30% higher in the normal hematocrit group than the low hematocrit group, although this was not statistically significantly different when the study was stopped. The incidence of thrombosis of vascular access sites was higher in the normal hematocrit group than in the low hematocrit. There were no differences in the rates of occurrence for all-cause hospitalization for all causes, nonfatal myocardial infarction, angina pectoris requiring hospitalization, congestive heart failure requiring hospitalization, coronary-artery bypass grafting, or percutaneous transluminal coronary angioplasty.

More recently, a large randomized, controlled trial in patients with CKD not on dialysis was also terminated early, with a significantly higher rate of composite events (death, MI, hospitalization for congestive heart failure without renal replacement therapy, and stroke) among subjects randomized to a target Hgb level of 13.0–13.5 g/dL compared to those randomized to a target Hgb level of 10.5–11.0 g/dL (a later protocol amendment changed the targets to 13.5 g/dL and 11.3 g/dL, respectively) (57). For unclear reasons, a mean Hgb level of only 12.6 g/dL was achieved in the higher target group. The risk for the single outcome events of death and CHF hospitalization approached being statistically significantly greater ($p = 0.07$) in the higher Hgb group. Other studies have also shown either no benefit or a significant trend towards increased risk for some outcomes when Hgb levels are normalized with ESA therapy in CKD patients (58–60). Thus, until further analysis and information becomes available, most ESA-treated patients with CKD should have their Hgb levels maintained above 11.0 g/dL but below 13.0 g/dL, and perhaps even lower. A recent FDA alert, issued after two recently published CKD studies (57, 58), advised adherence to prescribing information for currently available ESAs recommending that the target hemoglobin be maintained in the range of 10–12 g/dL (http://www.fda.gov/cder/drug/InfoSheets/HCP/RHE_HCP.htm).

Conclusion

Anemia and CKD are both common underrecognized and undertreated conditions with significant effects on morbidity and mortality in the elderly. Recognizing the presence of CKD by determination of eGFR rather than relying on whether a serum creatinine concentration is "normal" or not is of paramount importance in the elderly. Elderly patients with CKD and anemia should have a thorough evaluation for causes other than, or in addition to, their CKD; often iron deficiency or other conditions will be found to be present also. Once these other treatable conditions are corrected, appropriate therapy with epoetin or other ESAs should be offered when appropriate, adhering to recommended treatment and monitoring guidelines.

References

1. Izaks GJ, Westendorp RG, Knook DL: The definition of anemia in older persons. *JAMA* 281:1714–1717, 1999
2. Chaves PH, Xue QL, Guralnik JM, Ferrucci L, Volpato S, Fried LP: What constitutes normal hemoglobin concentration in community-dwelling disabled older women? *J Am Geriatr Soc* 52:1811–1816, 2004
3. Eschbach JW: The anemia of chronic renal failure: pathophysiology and the effects of recombinant erythropoietin. *Kidney Int* 35:134–148, 1989
4. Stiveleman J, Fishbane S, Nissenson AR: Erythropoietin therapy in renal disease and renal failure, in *The Kidney*, edited by Brenner B, 7th ed, Philadelphia, PA, Saunders, 2004, pp 2539–2561
5. KDOQI Clinical Practice Guidelines and Clinical Practice Recommendations for anemia in chronic kidney disease. *Am J Kidney Dis* 47:S11–145, 2006
6. Lindeman RD, Tobin J, Shock NW: Longitudinal studies on the rate of decline in renal function with age. *J Am Geriatr Soc* 33:278–285, 1985
7. Nicoll SR, Sainsbury R, Bailey RR, King A, Frampton C, Elliot JR, Turner JG: Assessment of creatinine clearance in healthy subjects over 65 years of age. *Nephron* 59:621–625, 1991
8. Fehrman-Ekholm I, Skeppholm L: Renal function in the elderly (>70 years old) measured by means of iohexol clearance, serum creatinine, serum urea and estimated clearance. *Scand J Urol Nephrol* 38:73–77, 2004
9. Rowe JW, Andres R, Tobin JD, Norris AH, Shock NW: The effect of age on creatinine clearance in men: a cross-sectional and longitudinal study. *J Gerontol* 31:155–163, 1976
10. US Renal Data System: USRDS 2005 Annual Data Report: Atlas of End-Stage Renal Disease in the United States. *Am J Kidney Dis* 47 (Suppl 1):S17–S268, 2006
11. Salive ME, Jones CA, Guralnik JM, Agodoa LY, Pahor M, Wallace RB: Serum creatinine levels in older adults: relationship with health status and medications. *Age Ageing* 24:142–150, 1995
12. Cumming RG, Mitchell P, Craig JC, Knight JF: Renal impairment and anaemia in a population-based study of older people. *Intern Med J* 34:20–23, 2004
13. Levey AS, Bosch JP, Lewis JB, Greene T, Rogers N, Roth D: A more accurate method to estimate glomerular filtration rate from serum creatinine: a new prediction equation. Modification of Diet in Renal Disease Study Group. *Ann Intern Med* 130:461–470, 1999
14. National Kidney Foundation: NKF-K/DOQI Clinical practice guidelines for chronic kidney disease: evaluation, classification, and stratification. *Am J Kidney Dis* 39 (Suppl 1): S1–S266, 2002
15. Cockcroft DW, Gault MH: Prediction of creatinine clearance from serum creatinine. *Nephron* 16:31–41, 1976

16. Verhave JC, Fesler P, Ribstein J, du Cailar G, Mimran A: Estimation of renal function in subjects with normal serum creatinine levels: influence of age and body mass index. *Am J Kidney Dis* 46:233–241, 2005

17. Lamb EJ, Webb MC, Abbas NA: The significance of serum troponin T in patients with kidney disease: a review of the literature. *Ann Clin Biochem* 41:1–9, 2004

18. Lamb EJ, Wood J, Stowe HJ, O'Riordan SE, Webb MC, Dalton RN: Susceptibility of glomerular filtration rate estimations to variations in creatinine methodology: a study in older patients. *Ann Clin Biochem* 42:11–18, 2005

19. Garg AX, Papaioannou A, Ferko N, Campbell G, Clarke JA, Ray JG: Estimating the prevalence of renal insufficiency in seniors requiring long-term care. *Kidney Int* 65:649–653, 2004

20. O'Riordan SE, Webb MC, Stowe HJ, Simpson DE, Kandarpa M, Coakley AJ, Newman DJ, Saunders JA, Lamb EJ: Cystatin C improves the detection of mild renal dysfunction in older patients. *Ann Clin Biochem* 40:648–655, 2003

21. Dharnidharka VR, Kwon C, Stevens G: Serum cystatin C is superior to serum creatinine as a marker of kidney function: a meta-analysis. *Am J Kidney Dis* 40:221–226, 2002

22. Van Den Noortgate NJ, Janssens WH, Delanghe JR, Afschrift MB, Lameire NH: Serum cystatin C concentration compared with other markers of glomerular filtration rate in the old old. *J Am Geriatr Soc* 50:1278–1282, 2002

23. Hsu CY, McCulloch CE, Curhan GC: Epidemiology of anemia associated with chronic renal insufficiency among adults in the United States: results from the Third National Health and Nutrition Examination Survey. *J Am Soc Nephrol* 13:504–510, 2002

24. Astor BC, Muntner P, Levin A, Eustace JA, Coresh J: Association of kidney function with anemia: the Third National Health and Nutrition Examination Survey (1988–1994). *Arch Intern Med* 162:1401–1408, 2002

25. McClellan W, Aronoff SL, Bolton WK, Hood S, Lorber DL, Tang KL, Tse TF, Wasserman B, Leiserowitz M: The prevalence of anemia in patients with chronic kidney disease. *Curr Med Res Opin* 20:1501–1510, 2004

26. van Ypersele de Strihou C: Should anaemia in subtypes of CRF patients be managed differently? *Nephrol Dial Transplant* 14 (Suppl 2):37–45, 1999

27. Guralnik JM, Eisenstaedt RS, Ferrucci L, Klein HG, Woodman RC: Prevalence of anemia in persons 65 years and older in the United States: evidence for a high rate of unexplained anemia. *Blood* 104:2263–2268, 2004

28. Weber JP, Walsh PC, Peters CA, Spivak JL: Effect of reversible androgen deprivation on hemoglobin and serum immunoreactive erythropoietin in men. *Am J Hematol* 36:190–194, 1991

29. Ershler WB, Sheng S, McKelvey J, Artz AS, Denduluri N, Tecson J, Taub DD, Brant LJ, Ferrucci L, Longo DL: Serum erythropoietin and aging: a longitudinal analysis. *J Am Geriatr Soc* 53:1360–1365, 2005

30. Kario K, Matsuo T, Kodama K, Nakao K, Asada R: Reduced erythropoietin secretion in senile anemia. *Am J Hematol* 41:252–257, 1992

31. Powers JS, Krantz SB, Collins JC, Meurer K, Failinger A, Buchholz T, Blank M, Spivak JL, Hochberg M, Baer A, et al.: Erythropoietin response to anemia as a function of age. *J Am Geriatr Soc* 39:30–32, 1991

32. Goodnough LT, Price TH, Parvin CA: The endogenous erythropoietin response and the erythropoietic response to blood loss anemia: the effects of age and gender. *J Lab Clin Med* 126:57–64, 1995

33. Artz AS, Fergusson D, Drinka PJ, Gerald M, Bidenbender R, Lechich A, Silverstone F, McCamish MA, Dai J, Keller E, Ershler WB: Mechanisms of unexplained anemia in the nursing home. *J Am Geriatr Soc* 52:423–427, 2004

34. Joosten E, Van Hove L, Lesaffre E, Goossens W, Dereymaeker L, Van Goethem G, Pelemans W: Serum erythropoietin levels in elderly inpatients with anemia of chronic disorders and iron deficiency anemia. *J Am Geriatr Soc* 41:1301–1304, 1993

35. Carpenter MA, Kendall RG, O'Brien AE, Chapman C, Sebastian JP, Belfield PW, Norfolk DR: Reduced erythropoietin response to anaemia in elderly patients with normocytic anaemia. *Eur J Haematol* 49:119–121, 1992

36. Zauber NP, Zauber AG: Hematologic data of healthy very old people. *Jama* 257:2181–2184, 1987

37. Ble A, Fink JC, Woodman RC, Klausner MA, Windham BG, Guralnik JM, Ferrucci L: Renal function, erythropoietin, and anemia of older persons: the InCHIANTI study. *Arch Intern Med* 165:2222–2227, 2005

38. Culleton BF, Manns BJ, Zhang J, Tonelli M, Klarenbach S, Hemmelgarn BR: Impact of anemia on hospitalization and mortality in older adults. *Blood* 107:3841–3846, 2006

39. Li S, Foley RN, Collins AJ: Anemia and cardiovascular disease, hospitalization, end stage renal disease, and death in older patients with chronic kidney disease. *Int Urol Nephrol* 37:395–402, 2005

40. Kurella M, Chertow GM, Fried LF, Cummings SR, Harris T, Simonsick E, Satterfield S, Ayonayon H, Yaffe K: Chronic kidney disease and cognitive impairment in the elderly: the health, aging, and body composition study. *J Am Soc Nephrol* 16:2127–2133, 2005

41. Nissenson AR, Wade S, Goodnough T, Knight K, Dubois RW: Economic burden of anemia in an insured population. *J Manag Care Pharm* 11:565–574, 2005

42. Mody S, Boyce S, Moyneur E, Piech C: Economic impact of untreated anemia in non-dialysis chronic kidney disease (NDCKD) patients [abstract]. *J Am Soc Nephrol* 14:457A, 2003

43. Lefebvre P, Duh MS, Buteau S, Bookhart B, Mody SH: Medical costs of untreated anemia in elderly patients with predialysis chronic kidney disease. *J Am Soc Nephrol*, 2006

44. Eschbach JW, Abdulhadi MH, Browne JK, Delano BG, Downing MR, Egrie JC, Evans RW, Friedman EA, Graber SE, Haley NR, et al.: Recombinant human erythropoietin in anemic patients with end-stage renal disease. Results of a phase III multicenter clinical trial. *Ann Intern Med* 111:992–1000, 1989

45. Eschbach JW, Egrie JC, Downing MR, Browne JK, Adamson JW: Correction of the anemia of end-stage renal disease with recombinant human erythropoietin. Results of a combined phase I and II clinical trial. *N Engl J Med* 316:73–78, 1987

46. Macdougall IC: Recent advances in erythropoietic agents in renal anemia. *Semin Nephrol* 26:313–318, 2006

47. Agarwal AK, Silver MR, Reed JE, Dhingra RK, Liu W, Varma N, Stehman-Breen C: An open-label study of darbepoetin alfa administered once monthly for the maintenance of haemoglobin concentrations in patients with chronic kidney disease not receiving dialysis. *J Intern Med* 260:577–585, 2006

48. Ling B, Walczyk M, Agarwal A, Carroll W, Liu W, Brenner R: Darbepoetin alfa administered once monthly maintains hemoglobin concentrations in patients with chronic kidney disease. *Clin Nephrol* 63:327–334, 2005

49. Locatelli F, Del Vecchio L, Marai P: Clinical experience with darbepoetin-alfa (Aranesp). *Contrib Nephrol* 137:403–407, 2002

50. Macdougall IC: CERA (Continuous Erythropoietin Receptor Activator): a new erythropoiesis-stimulating agent for the treatment of anemia. *Curr Hematol Rep* 4:436–440, 2005

51. Shank WA, Jr., Balducci L: Recombinant hemopoietic growth factors: comparative hemopoietic response in younger and older subjects. *J Am Geriatr Soc* 40:151–154, 1992

52. Nicholas JC: A study of the response of elderly patients with end-stage renal disease to epoetin alfa or beta. *Drugs Aging* 21:187–201, 2004
53. Ali A, Juhoor N, Farmer B, Davenport D: Do elderly hemodialysis patients (>70 years) respond to erythropoietin (EPO) treatment? [abstract]. *J Am Soc Nephrol* 7:1436, 1996
54. Delano BG: Improvements in quality of life following treatment with r-HuEPO in anemic hemodialysis patients. *Am J Kidney Dis* 14:14–18, 1989
55. Moreno F, Aracil FJ, Perez R, Valderrabano F: Controlled study on the improvement of quality of life in elderly hemodialysis patients after correcting end-stage renal disease-related anemia with erythropoietin. *Am J Kidney Dis* 27:548–556, 1996
56. Besarab A, Bolton WK, Browne JK, Egrie JC, Nissenson AR, Okamoto DM, Schwab SJ, Goodkin DA: The effects of normal as compared with low hematocrit values in patients with cardiac disease who are receiving hemodialysis and epoetin. *N Engl J Med* 339:584–590, 1998
57. Singh AK, Szczech L, Tang KL, Barnhart H, Sapp S, Wolfson M, Reddan D: Correction of anemia with epoetin alfa in chronic kidney disease. *N Engl J Med* 355:2085–2098, 2006
58. Drueke TB, Locatelli F, Clyne N, Eckardt KU, Macdougall IC, Tsakiris D, Burger HU, Scherhag A: Normalization of hemoglobin level in patients with chronic kidney disease and anemia. *N Engl J Med* 355:2071–2084, 2006
59. Roger SD, McMahon LP, Clarkson A, Disney A, Harris D, Hawley C, Healy H, Kerr P, Lynn K, Parnham A, Pascoe R, Voss D, Walker R, Levin A: Effects of early and late intervention with epoetin alpha on left ventricular mass among patients with chronic kidney disease (stage 3 or 4): results of a randomized clinical trial. *J Am Soc Nephrol* 15:148–156, 2004
60. Levin A, Djurdjev O, Thompson C, Barrett B, Ethier J, Carlisle E, Barre P, Magner P, Muirhead N, Tobe S, Täm P, Wadgymar JA, Kappel J, Holland D, Pichette V, Shoker A, Soltys G, Verrelli M, Singer J: Canadian randomized trial of hemoglobin maintenance to prevent or delay left ventricular mass growth in patients with CKD. *Am J Kidney Dis* 46:799–811, 2005

Chapter 6

Anemia in Long-Term Care

Andrew S. Artz and Miriam Rodin

Long-Term Care

Long-term care refers to a heterogeneous spectrum of facilities and health-related services that range from home nursing services to residential care and skilled nursing facilities, so-called nursing homes. Although the services eligible for Medicare coverage are defined by CMS, the clinical and demographic mix in facilities, even of the same level of care, is highly variable. The shifting health care environment has led to a shift towards increasing acuity in skilled facilities and rising levels of dependency in nonskilled assisted and supported living facilities and housing. In general, nursing homes provide two kinds of reimbursable Medicare service: subacute rehabilitation and skilled nursing. In both instances, admission to a nursing facility must have occurred within 30 days of hospitalization. It represents both the absence of adequate home supports and an illness-related decline in functional status. The goal is to return the patients to their previous level of function. However some proportions are never able to return to unsupported living. Increasingly, nursing homes have become the site of terminal care for patients without the resources for home hospice. Patients who are not Medicare eligible or have stayed beyond the 90 period must have another payor, usually it is Medicaid, some are self-pay.

Thus, the nursing home describes a transient and variable population. National figures support dividing this population into short-stay and long-stay residents. Indeed, the quality indicators reporting system that tracks nursing home performance distinguishes between long-term and short-term residents who totaled about 1.6 million people among greater 2 million admissions to nursing home. The average length of stay for current (1999) residents in nursing facilities was 892 days, or about 2½ years. Medicaid was the principle payor for long-stay residents. Short-stay residents are defined as those within the 90-day Medicare coverage period (1). Of patients discharged during the 1999 survey year, the average length of stay was 272 days, or about 8 months. Most of these residents over the age of 65 still required ADL assistance at the time of discharge. (DHHS, NCHS, CDCP. The National Nursing Home Survey 1999 Summary. June 2002. Vital and Health Statistics Series 13. Number 152). Thus, any nursing home admission and long-term residence in a care facility suggests an overall poor performance status. Most previous studies of anemia in nursing homes have selected these residents for study. They are reasonably stable and likely to remain so for the term of a study. As well, they reside in a setting in which multiple comorbid conditions interact with functional status and functional status is under continuous observation.

Anemia Prevalence

Indirect Measurement

As in other settings, anemia prevalence depends on the population and anemia definition. Estimates of anemia ascertained by ICD codes (280–284) have suggested a very low frequency. In the 1999 National Nursing home survey, only 2.4% of residents carried a diagnosis of anemia (ICD codes 280–284) (http://www.cdc.gov/nchs/data/series/sr_13/sr13_152.pdf). Examining the minimum data set (MDS) and anemia chart diagnoses, an 18.8% prevalence was reported among 43,510 NH residents 65 years and older in Missouri (2).

Direct Measurement

Direct measures of hemoglobin (Hb) concentration have shown a remarkably high prevalence of anemia in nursing homes, and underscore the limitations of using billing codes or chart history for anemia ascertainment. Direct measures may still be difficult to interpret. A series of reports indicated anemia prevalence of around 40% (3–9). Most of these studies were single institutional, included more than long-term care residents, and employed different Hb thresholds, accounting for extremely variable estimates of prevalence. For example, in a multilevel geriatric complex in Israel, in which 56% of residents were identified as "Nursing Home," anemia prevalence was 31% (9).

Most recent studies have employed the World Health Organization (WHO) threshold to define anemia of Hb < 13 g/dL for men and <12 g/dL for women (10). Although this threshold has been widely criticized (11, 12) based upon an association of adverse outcomes with higher Hb concentration, the WHO criteria remain useful to compare anemia prevalence in different studies. Using a standard definition may also allow anemia prevalence to serve as a surrogate for average Hb concentrations, assuming similar Hb distributions in the population. One may generally assume a lower average Hb concentration in the presence of higher anemia prevalence. Ania Lafuente (13) reported anemia prevalence of 36% for males and 44% for females upon nursing home admission in 198 subjects by WHO criteria. In 441 female nursing home residents aged 61–104, 49.7% had anemia by WHO criteria and mean Hb was 11.9 g/dL (14).

Table 6.1 shows the results of two recent multi-institutional studies by the National Geriatrics Research Consortium (NGRC) (15) and the RESTORE study (16). Both surveys measured anemia point prevalence using the WHO criteria among long-stay nursing home residents. The NGRC reported a 48% anemia prevalence among 900 long-stay residents in five facilities compared with anemia prevalence of 59.6% among 6,200 residents of 372 LTCF in the RESTORE analysis. The vast majority of

Table 6.1. Prevalence of anemia in the nursing home

	NGRC, 2004(15)	RESTORE(16)[a]
Sample size	900	6200
Facilities	5	372
Age, median	79	83
≥65 years	87%	100%
Female	63%	70%
Anemia		
Hemoglobin, mean (g/dL)	11.9 female	11.8 (total)
	12.9 male	
Prevalence[b]	48%	60%
Hb < 10 g/dL	11%	13%

NGRC, National geriatrics research consortium.
[a]Robinson et al, unpublished data.
[b]WHO criteria of Hb < 13 g/dL for men and <12 g/dL for men.

anemia was due to relatively modest Hb reductions, 11–13% of anemias had an Hb concentration <10 g/dL. The differences in anemia prevalence likely relate to study inclusion criteria. Both studies attempted to capture chronic long-term care residents and excluded acute rehabilitation patients, those having poor prognosis such as terminal illness diagnosis and dialysis patients as they are almost universally anemic if not on treatment. The NGRC did not exclude younger residents. Thus, 13% of residents were less than 65 years of age whereas RESTORE only included those 65 years and older. The median age for the NGRC was 79 years compared to 83 years in RESTORE. Since advancing age is associated with lower Hb and higher anemia prevalence (17–21), age differences may account for the higher anemia prevalence in RESTORE. The extent to which other factors impacted the anemia prevalence is not known.

The combination of these two studies demonstrates a 50% or greater anemia prevalence in older long-term care residents. This prevalence exceeds the estimated prevalence of anemia of 20–25% in community dwelling adults 85 years and over (21), older than the median age in the nursing home studies. Therefore, older age does not entirely account for the high prevalence of anemia in long-term care.

While anemia may be underappreciated as suggested by chart diagnosis and ICD coding, most residents will have an Hb available documenting anemia status. In the RESTORE analysis, exploring centrally and electronically available data, 2,107 of 10,315 (20.4%) did not have an Hb value. In contrast, only 2.7% (25/934) from the NGRC survey directly examining the chart record lacked an Hb measurement over the 6-month ascertainment period. It is likely that most long-term care residents have an Hb measure that would permit determining anemia status.

Adverse Outcomes

An emerging body of literature supports a strong and consistent association of anemia with adverse outcomes in community dwelling older adults including decreased physical performance (22), decreased mobility (23), decreased cognition (20), increased falls (24), increased hospitalization (12, 25), and increased mortality (12, 20, 25–28). Further, the adverse association occurs at mildly low Hb concentrations, often 2 g/dL above the WHO threshold for anemia.

To the extent that the adverse outcomes apply to older long-term care residents, the anemia may constitute an additional adverse prognostic factor. The few studies that examine the association of anemia with adverse among nursing home residents have lacked adequate power for appropriate adjustment for confounding factors, including comorbidity. Nevertheless, the data suggest the trend for older nursing home residents is similar to that seen in community-dwelling elderly.

Functional Status

A Spanish study reported an association between anemia on nursing home admission and decreased functional ability in men but not women (13). Dharmarajan and colleagues suggested an association between falls and anemia in 145 older adults admitted to hospitals for hip fracture (29). The sample included both nursing home and community–dwelling elderly. Anemic individuals suffered more falls than nonanemic individuals (30% versus 13%; $P = 0.028$).

Hospitalization

In an unadjusted analysis, the NGRC reported a 30% 6-month hospitalization rate for anemic nursing home residents compared to 15.8% for those without anemia (unadjusted odds ratio = 2.29, 95% CI 1.62–3.22). Hospitalization occurred in 55% for the subset having an Hb $\leq$ 10 g/dL. Very similar results have been observed in community-dwelling older adults. In a sample of community-dwelling elderly, multivariable adjusted RR for hospitalization was estimated at (HR, 2.16; 95% CI, 1.88–2.48) and a "dose response" for relationship for lower Hb values were associated with greater risk for hospitalization (12).

Mortality

Anemia may portend for higher mortality long-term care. In nursing home residents without heart disease, the 1-year mortality among women with and without anemia was similar at 8.1% and 8.5%, respectively. However, among those with heart disease, anemia was associated with a mortality of 27.9% compared to nonanemic residents of 13.1% ($P = 0.016$) (14). Kikuchi et al. (30) compared 63 long-term care residents having an Hb < 11 g/dL to matched controls and assessed 5-year survival. Anemia was associated with an increased risk of death (OR = 4.29; 95% CI, 3.55–5.12). Finally, among 43,510 residents 65 years or older across 522 facilities, anemia by chart diagnosis (rather than direct measurement) was associated with higher mortality at 1 year (2). After adjustment for functional status (i.e., ADLs), anemia was not statistically significantly associated with survival. At least six studies have shown an independent association between increased mortality and anemia in older community-dwelling adults, further supporting anemia as a negative prognostic marker (12, 20, 25–28).

Etiology

Anemia in older adults almost always represents an acquired condition. The contribution of hemoglobinopathies has not been described and could vary with the ethnic population of individual nursing homes. The importance of evaluating anemia in older adults to identify underlying conditions has long been appreciated. The appropriate evaluation hinges on knowledge of the most likely diagnoses in older adults. Studies precisely ascertaining the cause of anemia in the elderly remain limited and descriptive data of the spectrum of anemia in long-term care populations are sparse. Two issues further hamper definitive conclusions regarding anemia etiology – the lack of gold standard definitions and difficulty in accounting for multifactorial disease. We present observational data on the diagnostic and associated characteristics of anemia in LTC studies.

Iron Deficiency

Iron deficiency anemia is relatively common and easily diagnosed in most cases. Iron deficiency frequently results from chronic blood loss, although diminished iron absorption may contribute. The strong association between gastrointestinal lesions and malignancy leading to chronic blood loss and iron deficiency anemia underscores the importance of identifying iron deficiency (31, 32). Therefore, the anemia work-up for nursing home residents requires a working knowledge of the diagnostic armamentarium for iron deficiency. Numerous tests may be employed to diagnose iron deficiency anemia including red blood cell microcytosis, low serum iron, high total iron binding capacity, low iron saturation, low serum ferritin, elevated soluble transferrin receptor, and lack of iron stores on a bone marrow evaluation.

Serum ferritin is the most reliable and practical test to diagnose iron deficiency in the nursing home. A serum ferritin below the lower limit of the reference range confirms iron deficiency. However, as an acute phase reactant, serum ferritin may be in the normal range in older adults despite iron deficiency. Thus, raising the threshold of serum ferritin to <40 or 50 ng/mL greatly enhances sensitivity but maintains excellent specificity to render a diagnosis of iron deficiency (33, 34). Serum ferritin enables a more accurate diagnosis than serum iron, total iron binding capacity, and/or iron saturation which are more affected by intercurrent illness and nutritional states. While bone marrow evaluation represents an excellent method of determining iron stores, the need for referral and an invasive procedure limits the applicability in long-term care. Soluble transferrin receptor holds promise to diagnose iron deficiency in presence of inflammation (when the ferritin may be misleading), but it has not yet been proven to improve test performance in older persons and may not be readily available in contract labs servicing nursing homes.

Several early studies, without the use of serum ferritin, suggested a high frequency of anemia due to iron deficiency. Using a response to iron therapy as the gold standard, Kalchthaler reported 42% of residents had iron deficiency (6). Chen and colleagues examined red cell parameters and iron studies and concluded a 40% prevalence of iron deficiency among anemic long-term care residents (5).

The NGRC study randomly selected anemic nursing home residents to undergo a thorough and prospective anemia evaluation (35). Table 6.2 summarizes the findings. In this trial, after informed consent, a comprehensive evaluation of anemia etiology was performed in a random subset of anemic residents. In this small sample, iron deficiency accounted for 23% (14/60) of anemias, using a threshold of serum ferritin <50 ng/mL. Only 29% of subjects categorized as iron deficient by ferritin level anemia had microcytosis, highlighting the limitations of using microcytosis to identify iron deficiency anemia. Thus, a normocytic anemia should not preclude evaluation for iron deficiency. Kikuchi and colleagues examined bone marrow iron stores at autopsy of nursing home residents and found low iron stores in four (14%) of anemic residents. These data suggest that while iron deficiency occurs in the nursing home, the frequency is possibly lower than generally believed. Studies in noninstitutionalized older adults have also found about 20% of anemia attributable to iron deficiency lending further validity to the lower estimates (21). These studies may well miss cases that have been recognized and treated and may therefore underestimate the number of cases.

Iron supplementation affords a relatively simple opportunity for anemia correction depending on the underlying disease. The decision to undertake upper and lower endoscopy, with the attendant discomfort and difficulty of preparation for disabled or confused patients should be made in the context of the patients overall quality of life and estimated remaining life expectancy. There are no studies available that have reported on underlying causes of iron deficiency in older long-term care residents.

Anemia of Chronic Disease/Inflammation

The central role of inflammation in the pathophysiology of anemia of chronic diseases has long been appreciated (36) and may be better thought of as "anemia of chronic inflammation." ACI is a hypoproliferative anemia characterized by low serum iron and low to normal iron binding capacity. Standard laboratory studies do not accurately permit a diagnosis of ACI. Hepcidin, a hepatically synthesized peptide, is the primary regulator of iron homeostasis. Studies of hepcidin have helped unravel the link between

Table 6.2. Characteristics of anemia by etiology in the nursing home $N = 60$ (adapted from (35))[a]

Type	Hb	EPO	MCV	Ferritin	IL-6	Alb	CRP
Units	g/dL	mIU/mL	fL	ng/mL	pg/mL	g/dL	mg/dL
Ref	11.5–15.0	4.2–27.8	80–98	10–291		3.5–4.8	0–4.9
IDA ($n = 14$)	10.6 ± 1.1	29.0 ± 16.2	85.4 ± 7.0	22.5 ± 14.5	6.6 ± 2.7	3.7 ± 0.5	10.1 ± 15.4
ACD ($n = 8$)	11.0 ± 1.5	20.3 ± 7.6	93.1 ± 3.4	167.4 ± 79.1	44.3 ± 72.4	3.6 ± 0.4	36.9 ± 35.5
IA[b] ($n = 27$)	10.8 ± 1.0	14.6 ± 7.3	92.3 ± 5.9	201.6 ± 195.6	8.5 ± 7.8	3.6 ± 0.3	6.0 ± 5.0
Other ($n = 5$)	10.0 ± 1.2	13.4 ± 1.6	87.0 ± 9.3	356.0 ± 577.1	98.0 ± 106.8	3.6 ± 0.3	41.1 ± 68.7
CRI ($n = 6$)	11.5 ± 0.8	12.5 ± 4.2	89.5 ± 6.5	177.8 ± 215.9	7.5 ± 1.4	3.9 ± 0.3	8.3 ± 5.6
All ($n = 60$)	10.7 ± 1.1	18.6 ± 11.6	90.1 ± 6.7	166.9 ± 233.6	19.0 ± 41.0	3.7 ± 0.4	13.6 ± 25.7

SD, standard deviation; IDA, iron deficiency anemia; ACD, anemia of chronic disease/chronic inflammation; CRI, chronic renal insufficiency (estimated GFR < 30 ml/min); IA, idiopathic anemia (a.k.a. "unexplained" anemia); Hb, hemoglobin; EPO, erythropoietin; MCV, mean corpuscular volume; IL-6, interleukin-6; Alb, Albumin; CRP, c-reactive protein.
[b]No etiology of anemia uncovered.

inflammation and anemia. Inflammatory cytokines such as interleukin-6 increase hepcidin expression. Hepcidin impairs intestinal iron absorption and release from the reticulo-endothelial system promoting a hypoproliferative, hypoferremic anemia consistent with the clinical diagnosis of anemia of chronic disease/inflammation (37, 38). Hepcidin holds promise as a diagnostic aide for anemia of chronic disease/inflammation but is not available outside of research laboratories. At present, anemia of chronic disease/inflammation is probably best diagnosed by the presence of an inflammatory comorbid disease (e.g., chronic infection, collagen vascular disease, cancer), supportive laboratory findings, and elimination of alternative causes. In the absence of consensus diagnostic criteria, anemia of chronic disease accounted for 66% of anemia in one study of a mixed sample of older adults in a large facility (9). The prevalence of 66% was considerably greater than prior reports in community-dwelling or hospitalized elderly (21, 39). In the NGRC study, ACD was diagnosed only after exclusion of iron, B12, folate, and CKD, and with this definition occurred in only 8/60 (13%) (35). Multifactorial etiologies were not considered. The high levels of proinflammatory cytokines (i.e., C-reactive protein and interleukin-6) in subjects having anemia of chronic disease/inflammation compared to other anemic subjects supports the NGRC classification scheme that required the presence of an inflammatory comorbid condition (see Table 6.2 and Fig. 6.1).

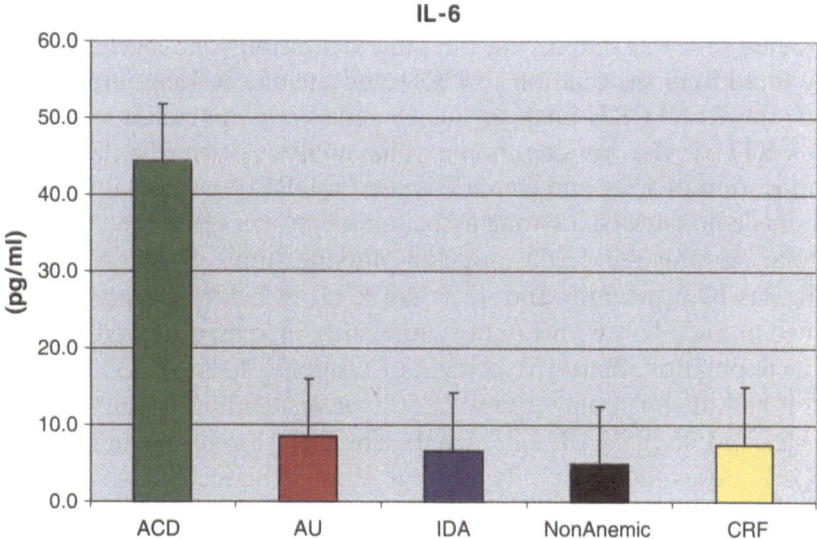

Fig. 6.1. Interleukin-6 (IL-6) levels by anemia etiology in the nursing home. ACD, anemia of chronic disease/inflammation; AU, anemia unexplained; IDA, iron deficiency anemia; CRF, chronic renal failure

Vitamin B12 and Folate Deficiencies

Deficiencies of vitamin B12 and folate remain important easily treated causes of anemia. However, they appear to be uncommon in skilled nursing facilities. Chernetsky and colleagues (9) suggested a prevalence of <5%. In the more recent NGRC analysis, no resident had low B12 or folic acid and anemia (35). One may postulate this relates to the wide use of multivitamin supplements in nursing homes. The higher prevalence in community-dwelling elderly indicates that identification and treatment could also account for the low prevalence in nursing homes (21).

Chronic Renal Insufficiency (a.k.a. chronic kidney disease/CKD)

Renal insufficiency may cause anemia due to variety of mechanisms, although low serum endogenous erythropoietin (EPO) levels may be the most important. EPO is a glycoprotein hormone produced by the kidney in response to anemia or hypoxia, and serves as a survival factor for erythroid progenitors. Even mild reductions in glomerular filtration rate (GFR) are associated with anemia (40). Attributing anemia due to CKD requires employing a GFR threshold below which any anemia will be considered caused by CKD. Most studies in older persons have used an estimated GFR of less than 30 mL/min (35, 41). The NGRC reported anemia due to CKD in 8% using a GFR < 30 mL/min by the Cockroft–Gault formula. In community-dwelling older adults, 8% of anemia has also been attributed to CKD employing the same definition (21). Designed specifically to address the relation to CKD and anemia in long-term care residents, the RESTORE analysis has extended our appreciation of anemia and CKD in the nursing home. The analysis used the four-variable Modification of Diet and Renal Disease (MDRD) to calculate GFR. The authors demonstrated a strong association between GFR < 60 ml/min and anemia. Among the 6,200 long-stay nursing home residents, the mean GFR was 69.6 mL/min and 43% had a GFR below 60 mL/min. CKD defined as a GFR < 60 mL/min significantly increased the risk of anemia in this population. Sixty-five percent of residents having CKD by this definition had anemia compared with 56% of residents without CKD (odds ratio [OR]: 1.47 [95% CI: 1.33, 1.63]). The inclusion of age in the formula for GFR raises the possibility that age alone explained the increased risk of anemia in CKD. Further analysis examined the association between CKD defined as GFR < 60 mL/min by 10-year age strata. Within each age strata the association between CKD remained significant. When elevated serum creatinine was used as a surrogate for CKD, the association with CKD and anemia persisted, independent of age. Other anemia etiologies were not considered, thus preventing clearly ascribing anemia to CKD. These data suggest renal function may affect Hb even in moderate renal insufficiency at a GFR between 30 and 59 mL/min.

Myelodysplastic Syndromes (MDS)

Myelodysplastic syndromes are a group of clonal hematopoietic stem cell disorders characterized by dysplasia and ineffective hematopoiesis (42). The diagnosis requires a bone marrow examination, which usually shows a paradoxical increase in cellularity despite peripheral pancytopenia because of a maturation block in hematopoietic stem cells (43). Although pancytopenia suggests MDS or another BM failure state, several types of MDS often present only with an isolated anemia. Since MDS most commonly occurs in older people, distinguishing anemia in older nursing home residents from MDS poses a major diagnostic challenge. The data are fairly limited because of the need to perform a bone marrow evaluation to accurately diagnosis MDS. Kikuchi and colleagues (30) assessed the bone marrow cellularity at autopsy in 29 cases with anemia (defined as a Hb < 11 g/dL), hypercellularity was not found, arguing against occult MDS in these patients. Other characteristic features of marrow dysplasia or chromosomal analysis were not assessed. In the NGRC study, three of 60 anemic residents had peripheral blood findings of macrocytosis (MCV of 100 fL), neutropenia, and/or thrombocytopenia. These findings were considered suggestive of MDS but bone marrow evaluation was not done. Whether this is an underestimate or overestimate of MDS remains unknown. It is reasonable to consider MDS in the presence of an unexplained pancytopenia or macrocytic anemia. With the availability of novel therapies, if the patients' treatment goals are consistent with the benefits and burdens of bone marrow biopsy, hematology consultation is warranted. Supportive care alone with erythropoiesis stimulating proteins (ESP) or transfusions is a viable alternative.

Unexplained Anemia (UA)

It has become increasingly appreciated that a sizeable fraction of anemia in older adults lacks an obvious etiology, ranging from 15 to 45% (21, 35, 39, 44). This "unexplained" anemia, sometimes described as "idiopathic" anemia or "senile" anemia, has blossomed as an area of active investigation. The necessary evaluation to exclude other causes before ascribing the anemia to the unexplained category has not been defined. The two major challenges are separating anemia of chronic disease/inflammation and how much additional testing must be performed before diagnosing UA. For example, should anemia absent another cause in a patient with coronary artery disease, congestive heart failure, and hypertension, but preserved renal function be considered UA or anemia of chronic disease/inflammation? Should a patient found to have UA undergo a more complete battery of tests such as testosterone level or gastrointestinal endoscopy even absent iron deficiency?

In the study by Chernetsky, 16% had UA but 66% were categorized as anemia of chronic disease (9). In the NGRC analysis, the most common diagnostic category of anemia was UA, present in 27/60 (45%). The mean MCV was 92 fL and mean Hb was 10.8 g/dL for UA. The high rate of UA occurred in a study with one of the most thorough anemia evaluations reported in older persons, suggesting the likelihood of considerable misclassification in studies reporting from other data sources. The NGRC study also demonstrated significantly higher CRP and IL-6 levels in the anemia of chronic disease/inflammation compared to UA (Fig. 6.1 and Table 6.2) supporting the concept that UA may be a separate and mechanistically distinct category of anemia from anemia of chronic disease/inflammation.

There may be overlap in the UA category with other conditions such as CKD. In the NGRC survey, anemia due to CKD was defined as an estimated GFR < 30 mL/min. The average serum creatinine was 1.0 mg/mL and the average GFR was 57 mL/min for UA. However, serum endogenous EPO levels were considerably lower than expected for the degree of anemia and lower than in nursing home residents having iron deficiency anemia (Fig. 6.2). Thus, inadequate endogenous EPO response to anemia may be a

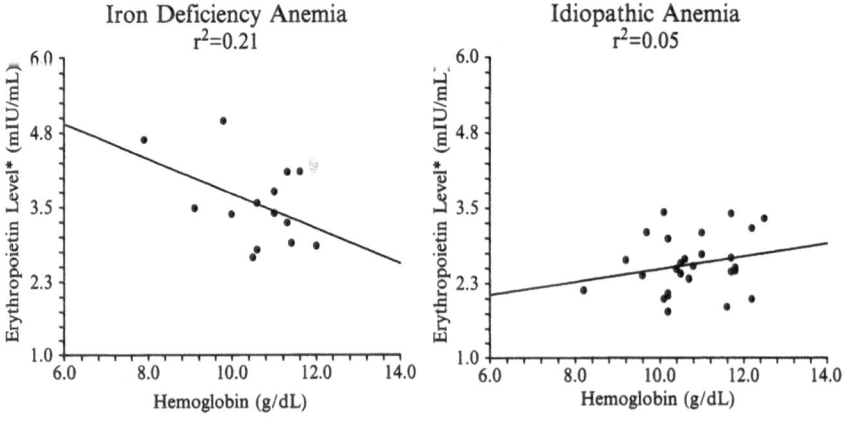

Fig. 6.2. Correlations between natural log transformed erythropoietin levels and hemoglobin comparing variances (r^2) of patients with iron deficiency anemia and idiopathic anemia

feature of UA and suggests that an endocrine renal defect contributes to this type of anemia. A blunted EPO response in older anemic subjects has been previously demonstrated in non-institutionalized elderly (45, 46).

The precise pathophysiology of UA will require further studies. Particularly relevant to nursing home residents is that some have postulated that protein-calorie malnutrition may be implicated in anemia in the long-term care setting (47, 48). In the NGRC study, the UA groups had a similar albumin and weight to the nonanemic group making severe malnutrition an unlikely cause of UA. Drug-induced bone marrow suppression should also be investigated in the long-term care setting where poly-pharmacy is common.

Anemia Evaluation in the Nursing Home

Based what is known about the common anemias observed in nursing homes, we suggest that an Hb and/or hematocrit be evaluated at some point on all nursing home residents, preferably on admission. We recommend an anemia work-up should the Hb meet WHO criteria of <13 g/dL for men and <12 g/dL for women or if the Hb is known to have fallen. The past medical history and physical examination should be assessed for relevant conditions such as chronic inflammatory diseases and infections. Medical implants such as cardiac valves and old joint prostheses secured with bone glue are not uncommon sources of hemolysis and sterile inflammation, respectively. The initial laboratory evaluation should include a complete blood count with red cell indices (e.g., MCV), serum creatinine, serum ferritin with or without serum iron and total iron binding capacity, and vitamin b12 and folate. GFR should be estimated based upon a formula accounting for age and weight. A reticulocyte count may be useful, especially if nutritional replacement has been initiated and especially to determine marrow response to anemia. However, one must recognize that most anemias in the nursing home are hypoproliferative and will likely have inappropriately low reticulocyte counts. Additional individual testing may be needed based upon signs and symptoms.

Anemia Treatment

For iron, B12, or folate deficiency, one should initiate supplementation. Except for iron deficiency, it remains unknown how likely or beneficial an etiologic investigation will be. For other anemias lacking a correctable chronic condition, three choices can be pursed: watchful waiting, red blood cell transfusions, or erythropoietin stimulating proteins (ESP). No controlled

Table 6.3. Use of anemia therapies in nursing home residents (%)

	NGRC (15)	RESTORE (16)[a]
Red blood cell transfusion	2.3	Nr
Erythropoietin stimulating protein[b]	2.9	2.6
Iron therapy	nr	19

nr, not reported.
[a]Robinson et al., unpublished data.
[b]Includes epoetin alfa and/or darbepoetin alfa.

data have evaluated the risk/benefit ratio of anemia therapies in the nursing home. Not surprisingly, ESP or red blood cell treatment appears quite infrequent in nursing home residents (Table 6.3) in <3% of residents. This underestimates the frequency of transfusion among nursing home residents, since few if any nursing homes can give transfusions, and severe anemia is generally discovered and treated in the course of an acute hospitalization. There would be no record of this in nursing home charts.

We generally reserve red blood cell transfusions for significant symptoms or when Hb falls below 8.0 g/dL and is at risk for further decline. Determining anemia-related symptoms can be difficult and often symptoms may only be identified after the Hb has improved from therapy. ESP approved in the United States include epoetin alfa (Procrit®, Epogen®) and darbepoetin alfa (Aranesp®). The primary indications are for anemia due to CKD or cancer chemotherapy. For the small number of residents receiving myelosuppressive cancer chemotherapy, ESP treatment can obviate red blood cell transfusions and enhance quality of life (49) when the Hb falls below 10–11 g/dL. The reduced marrow reserve in older adults may predispose to hematologic toxicity, such as anemia.

Anemia due to CKD is the most common etiology in long-term care residents for which ESP therapy may be entertained. While ESP therapy has found widespread use for anemia due to CKD (50), the risks and benefits in this population, particularly for residents not on dialysis and not receiving red cell transfusions remain unexplored. In light of the increased risk of thrombosis and hypertension associated with ESP in a population at increased danger for such events, caution must be exercised. Prescribing should be restricted to physicians experienced in the use and monitoring of ESP treatment. We generally will use an ESP for anemia due to CKD to obviate red blood cell transfusions, assuming all other etiologies have been excluded. We will consider ESP therapy for anemia of CKD if the Hb is < 10 g/dL, the patient can be monitored closely for complications, the patient or caregiver understand the risks, and a clear quality of life improvement can be measured. The issues of informed consent and caregiver training are more complex in a nursing home where patients may be cognitively compromised and rotating staff nurses makes continuity impractical from the point of view of in-service training. However, if we believe that ESP may improve the patient's functional status and quality of life, we are careful not to exceed 12 g/dL in light of the risk of increased complications at higher Hb concentrations (51, 52). Iron supplementation is frequently needed to prevent iron restricted erythropoiesis once on ESP treatment. We do not believe Hb improvement by itself, absent red blood cell transfusion dependence, is a sufficient justification for continuous ESP therapy in this setting. Interventional anemia trials in long-term care are sorely needed to establish evidence-based guidelines for future recommendations.

References

1. Konetzka RT, Norton EC, Sloane PD, et al. Medicare prospective payment and quality of care for long-stay nursing facility residents. *Med Care* 2006;44(3): 270–6.
2. van Dijk PT, Mehr DR, Ooms ME, et al. Comorbidity and 1-year mortality risks in nursing home residents. *J Am Geriatr Soc* 2005;53(4): 660–5.
3. Harant Z, Goldberger JV. Treatment of anemia in the aged: a common problem and challenge. *J Am Geriatr Soc* 1975;23(3): 127–31.
4. Barclay DV, Heredia L, Gil-Ramos J, et al. Nutritional status of institutionalised elderly in Ecuador. *Arch Latinoam Nutr* 1996;46(2): 122–7.
5. Chen LH, Cook-Newell ME. Anemia and iron status in the free-living and institutionalized elderly in Kentucky. *Int J Vitam Nutr Res* 1989;59(2): 207–13.
6. Kalchthaler T, Tan ME. Anemia in institutionalized elderly patients. *J Am Geriatr Soc* 1980;28(3): 108–13.
7. Salive ME, Cornoni-Huntley J, Guralnik JM et al. Anemia and hemoglobin levels in older persons: relationship with age, gender, and health status. *J Am Geriatr Soc* 1992;40(5): 489–96.
8. Sahadevan S, Choo PW, Jayaratnam FJ. Anaemia in the hospitalised elderly. *Singapore Med J* 1995;36(4): 375–8.
9. Chernetsky A, Sofer O, Rafael C, Ben-Israel J. Prevalence and etiology of anemia in an institutionalized geriatric population. *Harefuah* 2002;141(7): 591–4, 667.
10. World Health Organization. Nutritional anemias. Report of a WHO scientific group. *World Health Organ Tech Rep Ser* 1968;405: 5–37.
11. Spivak JL. Anemia in the elderly: time for new blood in old vessels? *Arch Intern Med* 2005;165(19): 2187–9.
12. Culleton BF, Manns BJ, Zhang J, et al. Impact of anemia on hospitalization and mortality in older adults. *Blood* 2006;107(10): 3841–6.
13. Ania Lafuente BJ, Fernandez-Burriel Tercero M, Suarez Almenara JL et al. Anemia and functional incapacity at admission to a geriatric home. *An Med Interna* 2001;18(1): 9–12.
14. De Maria R, Ripamonti V, Sandri R, et al. The negative prognostic synergism of anemia and heart disease in female nursing home residents. *Am J Cardiol* 2005;96(10): 1460–2.

15. Artz AS, Fergusson D, Drinka PJ, et al. Prevalence of anemia in skilled-nursing home residents. *Arch Gerontol Geriatr* 2004;39(3): 201–6.

16. Narayanan S, Critchlow C, Sciarra A, et al. Chronic Kidney Disease (CKD) associated anemia is common in elderly nursing-home residents. *J Am Soc Nephrol* 2005;16: 549.

17. Lesourd B, Decarli B, Dirren H. Longitudinal changes in iron and protein status of elderly Europeans. SENECA Investigators. *Eur J Clin Nutr* 1996;50(Suppl 2): S16–24.

18. Nilsson-Ehle H, Jagenburg R, Landahl S, Svanborg A. Blood haemoglobin declines in the elderly: implications for reference intervals from age 70 to 88. *Eur J Haematol* 2000;65(5): 297–305.

19. Ershler WB, Sheng S, McKelvey J, et al. Serum erythropoietin and aging: a longitudinal analysis. *J Am Geriatr Soc* 2005;53(8): 1360–5.

20. Denny SD, Kuchibhatla MN, Cohen HJ. Impact of anemia on mortality, cognition, and function in community-dwelling elderly. *Am J Med* 2006;119(4): 327–34.

21. Guralnik JM, Eisenstaedt RS, Ferrucci L, et al. Prevalence of anemia in persons 65 years and older in the United States: evidence for a high rate of unexplained anemia. *Blood* 2004;104(8): 2263–8.

22. Penninx BW, Pahor M, Cesari M, et al. Anemia is associated with disability and decreased physical performance and muscle strength in the elderly. *J Am Geriatr Soc* 2004;52(5): 719–24.

23. Chaves PH, Ashar B, Guralnik JM, Fried LP. Looking at the relationship between hemoglobin concentration and prevalent mobility difficulty in older women. Should the criteria currently used to define anemia in older people be reevaluated? *J Am Geriatr Soc* 2002;50(7): 1257–64.

24. Dharmarajan TS, Avula S, Norkus EP. Anemia increases risk for falls in hospitalized older adults: an evaluation of falls in 362 hospitalized, ambulatory, long-term care, and community patients. *J Am Med Dir Assoc* 2006;7(5): 287–93.

25. Penninx BW, Pahor M, Woodman RC, Guralnik JM. Anemia in old age is associated with increased mortality and hospitalization. *J Gerontol A Biol Sci Med Sci* 2006;61(5): 474–9.

26. Chaves PH, Xue QL, Guralnik JM, et al. What constitutes normal hemoglobin concentration in community-dwelling disabled older women? *J Am Geriatr Soc* 2004;52(11): 1811–6.

27. Zakai NA, Katz R, Hirsch C, et al. A prospective study of anemia status, hemoglobin concentration, and mortality in an elderly cohort: the Cardiovascular Health Study. *Arch Intern Med* 2005;165(19): 2214–20.

28. Izaks GJ, Westendorp RG, Knook DL. The definition of anemia in older persons. *JAMA* 1999;281(18): 1714–7.

29. Dharmarajan TS, Norkus EP. Mild anemia and the risk of falls in older adults from nursing homes and the community. *J Am Med Dir Assoc* 2004;5(6): 395–400.

30. Kikuchi M, Inagaki T, Shinagawa N. Five-year survival of older people with anemia: variation with hemoglobin concentration. *J Am Geriatr Soc* 2001;49(9): 1226–8.

31. Coban E, Timuragaoglu A, Meric M. Iron deficiency anemia in the elderly: prevalence and endoscopic evaluation of the gastrointestinal tract in outpatients. *Acta Haematol* 2003;110(1): 25–8.

32. Joosten E, Ghesquiere B, Linthoudt H, et al. Upper and lower gastrointestinal evaluation of elderly inpatients who are iron deficient. *Am J Med* 1999;107(1): 24–9.

33. Joosten E, Van Loon R, Billen J, et al. Serum transferrin receptor in the evaluation of the iron status in elderly hospitalized patients with anemia. *Am J Hematol* 2002;69(1): 1–6.

34. Guyatt GH, Patterson C, Ali M, et al. Diagnosis of iron-deficiency anemia in the elderly. *Am J Med* 1990;88(3): 205–9.
35. Artz AS, Fergusson D, Drinka PJ, et al. Mechanisms of unexplained anemia in the nursing home. *J Am Geriatr Soc* 2004;52(3): 423–7.
36. Krantz SB. Pathogenesis and treatment of the anemia of chronic disease. *Am J Med Sci* 1994;307(5): 353–9.
37. Nemeth E, Rivera S, Gabayan V, et al. IL-6 mediates hypoferremia of inflammation by inducing the synthesis of the iron regulatory hormone hepcidin. *J Clin Invest* 2004;113(9): 1271–6.
38. Andrews NC. Anemia of inflammation: the cytokine-hepcidin link. *J Clin Invest* 2004;113(9): 1251–3.
39. Joosten E, Pelemans W, Hiele M, et al. Prevalence and causes of anaemia in a geriatric hospitalized population. *Gerontology* 1992;38(1–2): 111–7.
40. Hsu CY, McCulloch CE, Curhan GC. Epidemiology of anemia associated with chronic renal insufficiency among adults in the United States: results from the Third National Health and Nutrition Examination Survey. *J Am Soc Nephrol* 2002;13(2): 504–10.
41. Ble A, Fink JC, Woodman RC, et al. Renal function, erythropoietin, and anemia of older persons: the InCHIANTI study. *Arch Intern Med* 2005;165(19): 2222–7.
42. Heaney ML, Golde DW. Myelodysplasia. *N Engl J Med* 1999;340(21): 1649–60.
43. Bennett JM, Catovsky D, Daniel MT, et al. Proposals for the classification of the myelodysplastic syndromes. *Br J Haematol* 1982;51(2): 189–99.
44. Baraldi-Junkins CA, Beck AC, Rothstein G. Hematopoiesis and cytokines. Relevance to cancer and aging. *Hematol Oncol Clin North Am* 2000;14(1): 45–61, viii.
45. Kario K, Matsuo T, Kodama K, et al. Reduced erythropoietin secretion in senile anemia. *Am J Hematol* 1992;41(4): 252–7.
46. Carpenter MA, Kendall RG, O'Brien AE, et al. Reduced erythropoietin response to anaemia in elderly patients with normocytic anaemia. *Eur J Haematol* 1992;49(3): 119–21.
47. Abbasi AA, Rudman D. Observations on the prevalence of protein-calorie undernutrition in VA nursing homes. *J Am Geriatr Soc* 1993;41(2): pp. 117–121.
48. Rudman D, Feller AG. Protein-calorie undernutrition in the nursing home. *J Am Geriatr Soc* 1989;37(2): 173–83.
49. Rizzo JD, Lichtin AE, Woolf SH, et al. Use of epoetin in patients with cancer: evidence-based clinical practice guidelines of the American Society of Clinical Oncology and the American Society of Hematology. *Blood* 2002;100(7): 2303–20.
50. KDOQI Clinical Practice Guidelines and Clinical Practice Recommendations for Anemia in Chronic Kidney Disease. *Am J Kidney Dis* 2006;47(5 Suppl 3): S11–145.
51. Drueke TB, Locatelli F, Clyne N, et al. Normalization of Hemoglobin Level in Patients with Chronic Kidney Disease and Anemia. *N Engl J Med* 2006;355(20): 2071–84.
52. Singh AK, Szczech L, Tang KL, et al. Correction of anemia with epoetin alfa in chronic kidney disease. *N Engl J Med* 2006;355(20): 2085–2098.

Chapter 7

Myelodysplastic Syndromes and Aplastic Anemia: Pathologic and Immunologic Implications

John M. Bennett

The Myelodysplastic Syndromes (MDS) represent a heterogeneous group of bone marrow diseases of uncertain etiology characterized by a variable degree of cytopenias, predominantly but not exclusively anemia that is often macrocytic (1). The cytopenias reflect both ineffective hematopoiesis (marrow dysplasia or accelerated apoptosis) and increase in marrow leukemic blasts (2). In 85% of cases the marrow is normo to hypercellular but in 15% the marrow cellularity can be below 30% and, on occasion, below 15%, which raises the differential diagnosis with acquired aplastic anemia (3). In such instances it is necessary to depend on the morphologic identification of significant dysplasia of one or more of the myeloid cell lines or the identification of small clusters of blasts on a bone marrow biopsy. Over 50% of all cases occur in patients over the age of 70 years. Each year some 15,000 individuals will be diagnosed with MDS, although this may well be an underestimate. In a recent national survey of elderly patients with anemia (4) some 17% met the criteria for unexplained anemia and leucopenia or thrombocytopenia. This would amount to a prevalence of 163,000 individuals who might have MDS with a more careful evaluation.

Approximately 50% of patients have acquired chromosomal aberrations. The most common include; +8; del5q; −7 and 20q− (5). The median survival is about 3 years but can range from less than 6 months to over 10 years. Thirty percentage will progress to Acute Myeloid Leukemia. This is much more common when the initial percentage of blasts exceeds 5% compared to less than 5% blasts. Therefore, close to 70% of patients will suffer from complications of cytopenias without disease progression to AML. For these latter patients effective treatment of the marrow failure without the use of cytotoxic drugs should offer a more desired form of treatment, without the complications of chemotherapy.

There is strong evidence that in some cases MDS is the result of an intrinsic, presumably acquired, genetic defect in hematopoietic stem cells.

However, other patients clearly have an autoimmune basis for their disease, since clinically MDS may be associated with other autoimmune disorders and laboratory evidence has documented oligoclonal t-cell patterns in upwards of 50% of patients tested (6).

Aplastic Anemia

There is no' reason to provide an extensive discussion of Aplastic Anemia (AA) in this chapter, since there have been several excellent reviews recently (7). There are fewer than 1000 cases diagnosed each year. There are several age peaks, with about 20% associated with congenital/familial disorders such as Fanconi's anemia and dyskeratosis congenital. In contrast to MDS there is a strong link to viral infections such as Hepatitis virus.

About 50% have an association with PNH and a mutated PIG-A gene (8). These clones can be detected by flow cytometry but rarely progress to classical hemolysis or thrombosis.

In contrast to the marrows of the majority of patients with MDS the bone marrows are routinely very hypocellular (below 20% cellularity) with a marked decrease in hematopoietic precursor cells (CD34). In addition to severe anemia, the neutrophils are below 500/cmm, platelets below 20,000/cmm, and reticulocyte count below 1%.

At the N.I.H. investigators have reported increased t-cell inhibitory activity suppressing hematopoiesis in MDS (9). These observations, identified by the selective use of the t-cell receptor (TCR) variable β chain, and the observation that CD8+ cytotoxic t cells (CTL) can suppress hematopoiesis in coculture, both suggest that a common mechanism may be operational in both patients with MDS and those with severe aplastic anemia (SAA). An additional syndrome that has been described in both AA and MDS has been the association with Large Granular Lymphocytic Leukemia (LGLL) (10).

Therapy

In AA the success of immunosuppression with antithymoctye globulin (ATG) often combined with cyclosporine has altered the natural history of this previously highly fatal bone marrow failure disorder (11). About 60% of patients are "responders" as defined by improved blood counts and many will survive over 5 years without undergoing allogeneic bone marrow transplantation (AlloBMT). Survival rates are much higher in children than in adults.

Some initial excitement was generated by reports from Brodsky et al. (12), recently summarized that reported 14 excellent responses in

19 patients with severe aplastic anemia, with 16 alive at 24 months of follow-up. However, others (13) have cautioned that long-term follow up indicates relapses, and the risk of cytogenetic progression is similar to what is noted with other immunosuppressive therapies.

For those who fail immune therapy AlloBMT can cure upwards of 75% (7). Matched unrelated BMTs are much less successful (14). Of interest is that MDS and AML evolves in about 15% of all patients, the vast majority occurring in those who do not undergo AlloBMT.

MDS

In order to select the most appropriate treatment scoring systems have been developed. The most popular one is The International Prognostic Scoring System (IPSS) which considers the percentage of bone marrow blasts, the number of cytopenias, and bone marrow cytogenetics to predict survival and the potential for progression to AML (15). Patients with untreated MDS are categorized into four IPSS prognostic risk groups – low, intermediate-1, intermediate-2, and high – with median survival times of 5.7, 3.1, 1.2, and 0.4 years, respectively.

Standardized response criteria in trials of MDS are essential to evaluate outcome of therapy, to refine treatment according to patient and disease characteristics, and to permit comparisons among clinical trials. In 2000, an International Working Group (IWG) of investigators proposed standardized response criteria for several purposes: (1) to resolve the difficulties with the variable definitions used to describe the quality and quantity of response, (2) to consider risk-based treatment goals, and (3) to identify clinically meaning-ful responses across MDS subgroups. The criteria also recognized alleviation of disease-related complications and improvements in quality of life (QOL) as important treatment goals. The IWG criteria have since been adopted in many clinical trials. Limitations of the IWG criteria were surfaced based on practical experience. Therefore, a revised proposal was developed and pub-lished recently in *Blood* which is much more practical (16).

The selection of therapy for MDS is based on the patient IPSS risk cat-egory, age, and performance status. Treatment goals range from managing cytopenias and improving QOL in lower-risk MDS to altering the natural history of disease in higher-risk MDS (17).

High-intensity therapies (intensive chemotherapy and stem cell transplan-tation) are generally reserved for patients in IPSS higher risk groups and have been associated with cures in some patients. Younger patients in lower-risk IPSS groups are sometimes also considered for allogeneic stem-cell trans-plants because of the favorable benefit:risk ratio. While they carry a high risk of treatment-associated morbidity and mortality, their aims are to alter the natural history of the disease (through induction of complete response) and to prolong progression-free survival (PFS) and overall survival. Five-year survival rates range from 35 to 70% depending on risk factors (18).

Cytogenetic responses help to establish the degree to which the natural history of MDS may be affected by therapy. Recently, low-intensity therapy with azacitidine or decitabine has also been shown to alter the natural history of MDS. This observation suggests that improving outcome in MDS may be obtained through means other than achievement of complete response (the currently accepted dogma).

Supportive care to manage cytopenias is a standard approach in lower-risk MDS or in patients with higher-risk MDS who cannot tolerate higher-intensity therapy. Many patients in lower-risk MDS succumb to the consequences of cytopenias without disease progression to acute leukemia. Patients with lower-risk MDS often become dependent on frequent red blood cell (RBC) or platelet transfusions and experience repeated infections, bleeding, and morbidity and mortality, all associated with reduction in health-related QOL. Some treatments in lower-risk MDS may improve blood cell counts, achieve transfusion independence, and QOL, but may not necessarily improve survival or PFS. The design and conduct of the azacitidine study predated the IWG criteria. The reported response rates were: CR 7%, PR 16%, improved 37%. In the FDA approval summary the response rates were: CR 6%, PR 10%, improved 19% (19).

Two recent trials of lenalidomide in lower-risk MDS used IWG criteria to assess cytogenetic response. In one trial, 12 of 20 patients (60%) with pretreatment cytogenetic abnormalities had cytogenetic responses, including 10 complete cytogenetic responses. Of 12 patients with 5q31.1 deletions, 10 had a cytogenetic response (83%), including 9 complete cytogenetic responses (75%). Cytogenetic responses occurred in patients who also had an erythroid response. Evaluation of cytogenetic response in this trial resulted in identification of a cytogenetic subset of MDS with 5q abnormalities that may be highly responsive to lenalidomide (20). This led to a multi-institutional trial of lenalidomide in 148 patients with lower-risk transfusion-dependent MDS and 5q deletions. In that study the HI-E rate was 65% and the complete cytogenetic response rate was 35% (21). Based on the results, lenalidomide was recently approved by the FDA for this indication (December 2005).

In patients with higher-risk MDS, treatment with another hypomethylating agent, decitabine, was associated with cytogenetic responses. Of the 115 patients with a known karyotype prior to treatment, 65 had abnormal metaphases, and clonal abnormalities were identified in 61. Major (complete) cytogenetic response was observed in 19 of the 61 patients (31%). Their median survival was 24 months compared with 11 months in patients who had persistent cytogenetic abnormalities despite treatment (22). These results illustrate the value of using standardized cytogenetic response criteria in both lower- and higher-risk categories.

As in AA, MDS can be successfully treated with cyclosporine (CsA) and antithymocyte globulin (ATG). Studies from the N.I.H. using ATG for MDS (23) were published several years ago. Since then many other investigators have reported improvement in cytopenias in MDS patients treated with fully immunosuppressive drugs. While it is clear that some patients respond to immunosuppression, overall response rates have varied widely (0–66%), but have not usually exceeded 30% (24). Part of this variation may be related to the differing criteria used to evaluate response, which have now been standardized by an international working group, but most of the variation probably reflects the diversity of the disease. Those most likely to respond have a modest transfusion burden, are young, with normal cytogenetics and a low percentage of marrow blasts. Trisomy 8, which has an intermediate survival according to the IPSS, was highly associated with response to immunosuppression (25). Older patients were less likely to respond and more likely to progress to acute leukemia (Sloand, EM, personal communication to the MDS Foundation, 2006).

These results which are shared with other treatments for MDS indicate a common pathology and physiology for older patients (age above 60 years). It is possible that there are, at least, two types of MDS, one being more associate with an immune assault against myeloid precursors in younger patients producing profound cytopenias that mimick AA, while MDS developing in older patients is characterized by a more pronounced malignant stem cell defect.

References

1. Bennett, JM, Catovsky, D, Daniel, M-T, et al. Proposals for the classification of the myelodysplastic syndromes. Br. J. Haem. 1982;51:189–199.
2. Parker, JE, Mufti, GJ. Excessive apoptosis in low risk myelodysplastic syndromes (MDS). Leuk. Lymphoma 2000;40:1–24.
3. Tuzuner, N, Cox, C, Rowe, J, et al. Hypocellular myelodysplastic syndrome: new proposals. Br. J. Haem. 1995;91:612–617.
4. Guralnik, JM, Ershler, WB, Schier, SL. Anemia in the elderly: a public health crisis in hematology. Amer. Soc. Education Program 2005;520–532.
5. Sole, F, Luno, E, Sanzo, P, et al. Identification of novel cytogenetic markers with prognostic significance in a series of 968 patients with primary MDS. Haematologica 2005;90:1168–1178.
6. Kochenderfer, JN, Kobayashi, S, Wieder, ED, Su, C, Molldrem, JJ. Loss of T-lymphocyte clonal dominance in patients with myelodysplastic syndrome responsive to immunosuppression. Blood 2002;100:3639–3645.
7. Young, NS, Calado, RT, Scheinberg, P. Current concepts in the pathophysiology and treatment of aplastic anemia. Blood 2006;108:2509–2519.

8. Ware, RE, Picken, CV, DeCastro, CM, et al. Circulating PIG-A mutant T lymphocytes in healthy adults and patients with bone marrow failure syndrome. Exp. Hematol. 2001;29:1403–1409.

9. Barrett, J, Saunthararajah, Y, Molldrem, J. Myelodysplastic syndrome and aplastic anemia: distinct entities or diseases linked by a common pathophysiology? Sem. Hematol. 2000;37:15–29.

10. Sauntharajah, Y, Molldrem, JL, Rivera, M, et al. Coincident myelodysplastic syndrome and T-cell large granular lymphocytic disease: clinical and pathophysiologic features. Br. J. Haematol. 2001;112:195–200.

11. Maciejewski, JP, Risitano, A, Kook, H, et al. Immune pathophysiology of aplastic anemia. Inter. J. Hem. 2002;76(Suppl 1):207–214.

12. Brodsky, RA, Jones, RJ. Aplastic Anemia. Lancet 2005;365(9471):1647–1656.

13. Tisdale, JF, Maciejewski, JP, et al. Late complications following treatment for severe aplastic anemia with high dose cyclophoaphamide: follow up of a randomized trial. Blood 2002;100:4668–4670.

14. Deeg, HJ, O'Donnell, M, Tolar, J, et al. Optimization of conditioning for marrow transplantation from unrelated donors with aplastic anemia after failure of immunosuppressive therapy. Blood 2006;108:1485–1491.

15. Greenberg, P, Cox, C, LeBeau, MM, et al. International scoring system for evaluating prognosis in myelodysplastic syndromes. Blood 1997;89:2079–2088.

16. Cheson, BD, Greenberg, PL, Bennett, JM, et al. Clinical application and proposals for the modification of the International working group response criteria in myelodysplasia. Blood 2006;108:419–425.

17. Greenberg, P. (chair). NCCN MDS guidelines. http://www.NCCN.org/profesionals/physicians, 2006.

18. Cutler, CS, Lee, SJ, Greenberg, P, et al. A decision analysis of alllogeneic bone marrow transplantation for myelodysplasia: delayed transplantation for low risk MDS is associated with improved outcome. Blood 2004;104:579–585.

19. Kaminskas, E, Farrell, AT, Wang, YC, et al. FDA drug approval summary: azacytidine for injecable suspension; a review. Oncologist 2005;10(3):176–182.

20. List, A, Kurtin, S, Roe, DJ, et al. Efficacy of lenalidomide in myelodysplastic syndromes. N. Engl. J. Med. 2005;352:549–557.

21. List, A, Dewald, G, Bennett, J, et al. Lenalidomide in the myelodysplastic syndromes with chromosome 5q deletion. N. Engl. J. Med. 2006;355:1456–1465.

22. Kantarjian, H, Issa, JP, Rosenfeld, CS, et al. Decitabine improves patient outcomes in MDS. Cancer 2006;106:1794 1803.

23. Molldrem, JJ, Leifer, E, Bahceci, E, et al. Antithymocyte globulin for treatment of the bone marrow failure associated with myelodysplastic syndromes. Ann. Intern. Med. 2002;137:156–163.

24. Killick, SB, Mufti, G, Cavenagh, JD, et al. A pilot study of antithymocyte globulin (ATG) in the treatment of patients with 'low-risk' myelodysplasia. Br. J. Haematol. 2003;120:679–684.

25. Sloand, EM, Mainwaring, L, Fuhrer, M, et al. Preferential suppression of trisomy 8 compared with normal hematopoietic cell growth by autologous lymphocytes in patients with trisomy 8 myelodysplastic syndrome. Blood 2005;106:841–851.

Chapter 8

Anemia and Cancer

Kaaron Benson, Lodovico Balducci, and Matti Aapro

Introduction

This chapter explores the management of anemia in older cancer patients. Cancer is a disease of aging: more than 50% of all malignancies currently occur in the 12% of the population aged 65 and over; by the year 2030 older individuals are expected to account for 20% of the population and 70% of all cancer cases (1). Though not unique of older individuals, anemia is a common manifestation of cancer, especially of advanced cancer (2). The elderly are expected to suffer disproportionately of cancer-related anemia, because cancer becomes more common with age and because age itself is a risk factor for anemia (1–3).

Anemia is detrimental to cancer patients, because it compromises patient well-being, and it may increase the complications and reduce the benefits of antineoplastic treatment (2). Anemia of chronic inflammation (ACI) and of chemotherapy are the most common forms of anemia in cancer patients and both respond to pharmacological doses of erythropoietin (2, 4). The availability of a number of synthetic erythropoiesis-stimulating factors (ESF) that mimic the action of erythropoietin has allowed the correction of anemia in the majority of cancer patients.

After reviewing the pathogenesis of anemia we will examine the consequences of anemia for the older cancer patients and the benefits and potential risks of treatment with ESF.

Causes and Mechanisms of Anemia in the Cancer Patient

Table 8.1 lists common causes of anemia in patients with cancer. Anemia of chronic inflammation is the most common form of anemia in cancer patients and in older individuals, as aging is a form of chronic and

Table 8.1. Causes of anemia in cancer patients

Common causes
- Anemia of chronic inflammation (ACI)
- Chemotherapy-induced myelosuppression
- Iron deficiency
- Myelophthisis

Other important causes
- Cobalamine deficiency
- Renal insufficiency
- Folate deficiency
- Autoimmune hemolytic anemia
- Microangiopathic anemia

progressive inflammation (3, 5, 6). Central to the pathogenesis of this form of anemia is a "relative erythropoietin deficiency" that involves inadequate production of erythropoietin for the degree of anemia, and increased resistance of erythropoietic precursors to erythropoietin (7–9). Undoubtedly, in older individuals, some degree of renal insufficiency may be responsible for the reduced erythropoietin response to anemia, as the glomerular filtration rate declines almost universally after age 65 (10). Increased concentration of circulating inflammatory cytokines, such as interleukin-6 (IL-6) or tumor necrosis factor (TNF) may blunt erythropoietin production as well as the sensitivity of the erythropoietic progenitors to erythropoietin (3) (Fig. 8.1). In older individuals, Ferrucci et al. (9) showed a biphasic effect of inflammatory cytokines on erythropoietin production: in the absence of anemia, increased concentration of inflammatory cytokines was associated with increased concentration of erythropoietin, and in the presence of anemia, with reduced erythropoietin concentration. Similar findings were reported by Ershler et al. (8) in older individuals followed in the Baltimore Longitudinal Study. The authors hypothesized that inflammatory cytokines initially stimulate the secretion of erythropoietin, and that eventually, due to the continuous stimulation, the ability of the organism to produce erythropoietin becomes exhausted. This hypothesis is supported by experimental observations that IL-6 stimulates the kidney secretion of erythropoietin (11). The higher levels of erythropoietin seen in nonanemic individuals may fail to rise the hemoglobin concentration to supra-normal levels, as the sensitivity of

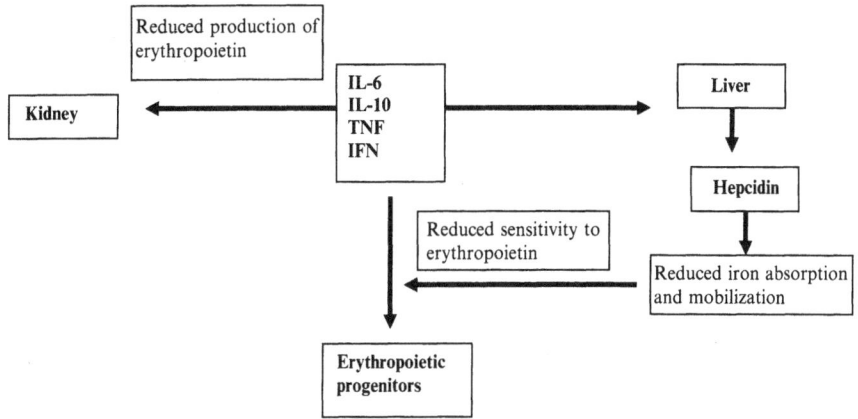

Fig. 8.1. Pathogenesis of anemia of Chronic Inflammation

erythropoietic progenitors to erythropoietin is blunted by the same inflammatory cytokines. Another consequence of chronic inflammation and more specifically of increased concentration of IL-6, is the increased hepatic production of hepcidin, a glycoprotein that prevents the mobilization of iron from the deposits as well as the intestinal absorption of iron (12). This fact explains while some cancer patients fail to increase their hemoglobin in response to erythropoietin, unless they are supplemented also with iron intravenously (13).

ACI is usually normochromic, normocytic but can, less commonly, be mildly hypochromic, and microcytic and typically is associated with low concentrations of iron, total iron binding capacity and soluble transferrin receptor (sTfR) in the circulation and increased levels of ferritin (4). The erythropoietin levels are variable but in general lower than those observed in iron deficiency for the same hemoglobin levels.

Chemotherapy-related anemia is hypoproliferative, macrocytic, and megaloblastic, and is due to the inhibition of DNA synthesis in erythropoietic precursors (2). Due to the concomitant presence of cancer, the majority of patients receiving cytotoxic chemotherapy also experience ACI, responsive to erythropoietin treatment.

The causes of iron deficiency in cancer patients include bleeding from cancer of the digestive tract and the endometrium, and bleeding from benign causes, such as diverticular disease of the colon, angiodysplasia, or polyps, all of which become more common with age.

Helicobacter pylori gastritis may also lead to iron deficiency as the microorganism utilizes the iron as a nutrient for its own growth, but the prevalence of this condition is unknown. It is reasonable, albeit not conclusively proven, to assume that some cases of iron deficiency in elderly individuals are nutritional, when a cause for iron loss is not found (14). Gastric atrophy may prevent the reduction of food-bound iron necessary for its absorption, and hepcidin may also hinder the absorption of iron (13). In its classical form iron-deficiency anemia is hypoproliferative, microcytic, and hypochromic, and is characterized by low circulating levels of iron and ferritin and increased levels of sTfR and total iron binding capacity (4).

The prevalence of cobalamin deficiency may be as high as 15% among individuals over 60 (15), due to failure to digest food-bound vitamin B12, which results from gastric atrophy. Oral cobalamin preparations may correct the deficiency in these patients (16). It should be emphasized that as many as 15% of patients with serum vitamin B12 levels between 180 and 300 pg/mL, which are considered normal, have functional vitamin B12 deficiency, as shown by increased circulating levels of methylmalonic acid and homocysteine (15–18). Unless it is associated with folate deficiency, cobalamin deficiency may not lead to anemia and its first manifestations in this case are neurological, including posterior column degeneration, peripheral neuropathy, and dementia (16).

Folate deficiency is common in patients with decreased food intake, including those with cancer of the head and neck and may be found among elderly individuals with low intake of leafy vegetables (17, 18).

Though more common in hematologic malignancies, myelophthisis may be observed in patients with solid tumors metastatic to the bones, especially breast cancer, prostate cancer, and small cell lung cancer. Myelophthisis may present as pancytopenia with an increased concentration of immature blood cells in the circulation (21).

Sarcopenia, a common manifestation both of cancer (22) and of frailty, may also contribute to the pathogenesis of anemia in older cancer patients, with reduced synthesis of proteins, including hemoglobin and erythropoietin (23).

Perhaps in the majority of cases the anemia of cancer is multifactorial and includes chronic inflammation, chemotherapy, and malnutrition. Correctable causes of anemia, including iron, folate, and cobalamin deficiency, hypothyroidism, and chronic renal disease should be investigated and managed. ESF are the mainstay of the management of ACI and chemotherapy-related anemia (2).

Complications of Anemia in Cancer Patients

The complications of anemia in the older cancer patient may include

- *Fatigue and functional dependence.* Fatigue is a feeling of tiredness unrelated to physical activity and not relieved by rest (24). It is the most common chronic symptom both of cancer and of chemotherapy, and is associated with serious consequences in the life of the patient and his/her caregivers, including reduction of working hours and even inability to work. Approximately 40% of cancer patients and 20% of their caregivers had to quit working or take leave from work because of the patient's fatigue (24). Fatigue is clearly related to anemia: correction of anemia relieves the fatigue of the majority of cancer patients and improves their quality of life (2). In older patients, anemia is also associated with increased risk of functional dependence, that is need of external help to carry on the basic activities of daily living (ADL) or the instrumental activities of daily living (IADL) (25–29). In older cancer patients fatigue is associated with functional dependence (30).
- *Chemotherapy-induced toxicity.* Anemia has been associated with increased risk of chemotherapy-induced toxicity (31–35). Anemia has a two-fold pharmacodynamic effect. Through hypoxia it may make normal tissues more susceptible to injury. In addition, anemia leads to a shrinkage of the volume of distribution of hydrosoluble agents, that are bound to red blood cells. In the presence of anemia the free concentration of these compounds in the circulation, and the risk of complications, may increase.
- *Reduced response to radiation therapy.* The response to radiotherapy of cancer of the upper airways, upper digestive tract, and the cervix was lower in anemic than nonanemic patients (2). Resistance to radiation therapy seemingly was mediated by tumor hypoxia, that prevented the formation of free radicals capable to damage the tumor DNA.
- *Impaired cognitive function.* Several lines of evidence indicate that anemia is associated with compromised cognitive function. In patients with end-stage renal failure, correction of anemia with ESF was associated with reduced incidence of dementia (36). Several studies reported higher prevalence of cognitive compromise among anemic than nonanemic elderly (37, 38). In a cohort study, Atti et al. (39) reported that anemia heralded the development of dementia over 3 years for individuals who were not demented (39). Likewise, the development of cognitive deficits in the course of adjuvant chemotherapy of breast cancer was more common in anemic patients (40).

- *Blood transfusion dependence and its associated risks.* Blood transfusions clearly serve a role in the management of severe anemia. Symptoms such as dyspnea on mild exercise or angina in patients with coronary artery disease respond promptly to blood transfusion. This treatment is associated with some risks, including transfusion-transmitted infections, transfusion reactions, transfusion-related immunomodulation (TRIM) with increased risk of tumor recurrence, and platelet refractoriness (41). Thanks to improvements in donor history questions and infectious disease marker testing, the risk of infections has been substantially reduced. Minor transfusion reactions, including urticaria and febrile nonhemolytic transfusion reactions, occur in about 0.5–1.0% of all transfusions, and while not harmful, can cause concern since they can mimic more serious reactions (41). TRIM has been deemed responsible for the poorer outcomes experienced by transfused patients as compared to those who had not been transfused (42). HLA and RBC alloimmunization is the consequence of multiple blood transfusions and may lead to delayed hemolytic reactions and to refractoriness to transfused platelets (43).
- *Adverse effects on longevity.* According to at least seven cohort studies (29, 44–49) anemia is an independent risk factor for mortality in individuals 65 and older, which represent 50% of all cancer patients (1).

Given the deleterious effects of anemia, and of blood transfusions, the ESF have represented a welcome addition to the management of anemia in older cancer patients. The effectiveness and risks of these compounds have been explored in a number of clinical trials.

Commercial Preparations of Erythropoietic Growth Factors

Currently available ESF include epoetin α, epoetin β (available only in Europe), and darbepoetin α (2). Darbepoetin α differs from epoetin α by the inclusion of glycosyl residues that prolong the half-life of the compound. Epoetin needs to be administered weekly, whereas darbepoetin may be administered every 3 weeks (50, 51). The activity of epoetin and darbepoetin appear similar and the main advantage of darbepoetin is less frequent administration.

Other erythropoietic stimulators are undergoing clinical trials. The CERA (Continuous Erythropoietin Receptor Activator), is a molecule of epoetin with a polymeric side chain that prolongs its half-life of several weeks (52) and may require less frequent administration than darbepoetin. A completely synthetic erythropoietic stimulator, Hematide, has been prepared and is undergoing early clinical experimentation (53).

Effectiveness and Risk of ESF in Cancer-Related Anemia

Trial designs. The management of the older cancer patients with ESF has been studied in three types of trials (2):

- Single arm trials in anemic patients aimed to establish whether improvement in hemoglobin resulted in reduction of blood transfusions and improvement in energy. The treatment was discontinued for hemoglobin levels around 12 g/dL.
- Randomized controlled trials in anemic patients aimed to establish whether improvement of hemoglobin was associated with better survival and response to chemotherapy in addition to improvement in quality of life and reduction in blood transfusions. In most of these trials ESF were discontinued for hemoglobin levels of 12 g/dL.
- Randomized controlled studies in anemic and nonanemic patients aimed to achieve and maintain normal hemoglobin levels, on the assumption that normal hemoglobin levels would have been beneficial both in terms of function, quality of life, treatment tolerance, and survival.

Effectiveness of the Treatment. We will address the benefits of ESF for each complication of anemia.

Fatigue. Treatment with epoetin α improved the anemia in 50–60% of patients with solid tumors who were followed longitudinally (54–56). The improvement in hemoglobin levels was associated with improved energy levels and quality of life and reduced incidence duration and severity of fatigue, irrespective of the status of the tumor. In other words, improvement of hemoglobin was beneficial to the quality of life of all patients, including those whose cancer had progressed. The maximal incremental improvement in energy was obtained when hemoglobin levels increased from 11 to 13 g/dL (24). These results were confirmed in subsequent randomized controlled studies (2, 57, 58).

Blood transfusions. Reduction of blood transfusions, thanks to ESF, was demonstrated in all randomized controlled studies. The average reduction in blood transfusions was approximately 30% (58).

Response to treatment and overall outcome. Treatment with ESF failed to improve survival, response to treatment, or chemotherapy-related toxicity in each of the randomized controlled studies. Patients enrolled in these studies had different types of tumors, at different stages and received different forms of treatment, so that it is difficult to draw definite conclusions related to survival (58).

Risk of functional dependence. This outcome is particularly relevant to older patients, for whom functional dependence is more common and more likely irreversible. One may infer a benefit of functional dependence from two studies. The Fatigue Coalition reported that fatigue was detrimental to the function of the patient and the caregiver (24). A decision analysis calculated that the cost of caring for older individuals was increased by anemia and the management of anemia with recombinant erythropoietin was cost-effective in these individuals (59).

Treatment complications. Three types of complications have been reported: autoimmune aplastic anemia (secondary to anti-erythropoietin antibodies), cardiovascular complications (including hypertension, venous, and arterial thrombosis), and increased rate of tumor growth.

Autoimmune aplastic anemia. This complication was described in 175 patients treated with epoetin α and β for anemia of chronic renal failure (60), was never reported in cancer patients, occurred exclusively in Europe, and appeared to be a manufacturing-related problem. Since standardized rules for preparation and handling of epoetin have been established, the incidence of this complication has decreased by 83%.

Cardiovascular complications. Concern about these complications, that have been well documented, prompted an Oncology Drug Advisory Committee (ODAC) conference involving all companies that produced recombinant erythropoietin (http://www.FDA.gov/ohrms/dockets/ac/04/slides/4037s2.htm). The conclusion of the conference participants was that the majority of these complications occurred in studies aimed to maintain normal levels of erythropoietin in cancer patients or in studies trying to increase the levels of erythropoietin too rapidly. As long as the currently recommended doses of erythropoietin were maintained and the treatment did not aim to levels of hemoglobin higher than 12 g/dL the treatment appeared safe and no special warning was needed.

Increased rate of tumor growth. The possibility of enhanced tumor growth was suggested in two published studies (61, 62), one in patients with cancer of the head and neck (61) and the other in patients with breast cancer (62) and was suggested in seven other studies reviewed by the ODAC conference. A recent meta-analysis of randomized controlled studies of ESF suggested a minor detrimental effect of these factors on survival (58). Definitive conclusions related to the risk of enhanced tumor growth could not be reached at the ODAC conference. The conference participants agreed that the overall risk, if present at all, was small enough that it did not erase the benefits of treatment. Also enhanced tumor growth appeared more prominent in studies aimed to maintain normal hemoglobin levels, but was negligible when hemoglobin levels were maintained around 12 g/dL.

An analysis of patients with head and neck cancer might have provided a clue to the potential risk of ESF in these patients (63). Some of the tumors, which were rich in erythropoietin receptors, experienced accelerated growth during treatment with ESF, whereas tumors poor in receptors did not experience growth stimulation. If this observation is confirmed, determination of erythropoietin receptors on the tumor may help select patients for ESF treatment.

Practical Issues Related to the Treatment with ESF

Which patients should be treated. According to the ASCO and NCCN guidelines (Table 8.2) (64) treatment should be initiated in all patients whose level of hemoglobin is lower than 10 g/dL. For hemoglobin levels between 10 and 12 g/dL the treatment should be initiated if the patient is symptomatic. In light of current knowledge these recommendations appear very reasonable and safe.

Table 8.2. Recommendation for treatment with epoetin in cancer patients

	ASCO	NCCN
Indications for starting treatment	Hb < 10 g/dL Hb < 12 g/dL in symptomatic patients	<11 g/dL
Response	Hb:1–2 g/dL	Hb:1 g/dL
Dose increment	No response 6–8 weeks	No response 8–12 weeks
Duration of treatment with increased dose	4–8 weeks	4–8 weeks
Discontinuance	No response after treatment with increased dose	No response after treatment with increased dose
Objective 12 g/dL	Hb: 12 g/dL	Hb:12 g/dL
Maintenance	D/C after reaching the objective or titrate dose to maintain Hb levels @ 12 g/dL	Titrate dose to maintain Hb levels @ 12 g/dL
Iron supplementation	No specific indication except for clear evidence of iron deficiency	Iron deficiency

When it is reasonable to stop the treatment? Generally it is recommended that treatment be discontinued for hemoglobin levels ≥12 g/dL. The increment in energy is lower when the hemoglobin rises above these levels and the risk of treatment complications increases.

What are the optimal doses? Common doses are 40,000 IU weekly for epoetin α and 300 ug/kg every 3 weeks for darbepoietin α. If after a month of treatment an increase in hemoglobin levels of at least 1 g/dL is not observed doses should be increased to 60,000 IU or 500 ug/kg, respectively. If no erythropoietic response is observed with these doses after 1 month, the treatment should be discontinued. Once hemoglobin levels ≥12 g/dL are obtained, maintenance treatment with reduced doses may be instituted. According to recent studies epoetin α may be effective at doses of 120,000 units every 3 weeks (65).

Should iron be administered together with erythropoietic growth factors? Iron deficiency should be corrected before therapy with recombinant erythropoietin. In patients with normal or increased iron stores, the addition of iron may be beneficial. A recent study randomized patients with cancer and chemotherapy-related anemia to receive no iron, oral iron, or intravenous iron (11). Whereas oral iron had no effect, intravenous iron was associated with a doubling of the erythropoietic response rate.

Erythropoietic Growth Factors and Red Blood Cell Transfusions: Effectiveness, Safety, and Cost Considerations

Red blood cell (RBC) transfusions have been the mainstay treatment of anemia until the introduction of ESF. The indications for RBC transfusions have been the treatment of symptomatic anemia. Patients commonly require blood transfusion when hemoglobin drops <7 or <8 g/dL or <10 g/dL when significant coexisting cardiac, pulmonary or vascular disease is present.

• The major advantage of erythropoietin over blood transfusions has been the maintenance of consistent hemoglobin levels, which resulted in consistent levels of energy and might have prevented life-threatening complications of anemia. When used according the ASCO and NCCN guidelines, erythropoietic growth factors appear safer than blood transfusions. Cremieux et al. (66) calculated that the monthly cost of treating a patient with epoetin α was similar to the cost of two monthly RBC transfusions. As only a fraction of patients treated with ESF would need two monthly blood transfusions according to the guidelines, it is clear that ESF increase the overall cost of cancer treatment.

This cost may be worthwhile when one considers the impact of fatigue on the indirect and intangible cost of managing cancer patients (67). This cost is particularly high for older individuals who are more susceptible to experience functional dependence as a consequence of anemia and fatigue.

Conclusions

In conclusion:

- In cancer patients anemia is responsible for fatigue and lower quality of life, poor therapeutic response, increased risk of chemotherapy related toxicity, and increased use of blood transfusions.
- In older individuals, anemia has been associated with reduced longevity, dementia, depression, and functional dependence.
- Correction of anemia with ESF has improved the function and quality of life of cancer patients, irrespective of their age, and reduced the use of blood transfusions.
- ESF appear safe when hemoglobin levels are maintained around 12 g/dL.
- Though costly, treatment with ESF appears to reduce the indirect and intangible cost of managing older patients with cancer.

References

1. Balducci L, Ershler WB: Cancer and ageing: a nexus at several levels. Nat Rev Cancer 2005;5:655–661.
2. Stasi R, Amadori S, Littlewood TJ, et al.: Management of cancer-related anemia with erythropoietic agents: doubts, certainties, and concerns. Oncologist 2005;10:539–554.
3. Balducci L: Anemia and aging or anemia of aging? Cancer Treatm Res 2007, in press.
4. Weiss G, Goodnough LT: Anemia of chronic disease. N Engl J Med 2005;352:1011–1023.
5. Maggio M, Guralnik JM, Longo DL, et al.: Interleukin-6 in aging and chronic disease: a magnificent pathway. J Gerontol A Biol Sci Med Sci 2006; 61(6):575–584.
6. Ferrucci L, Corsi A, Lauretani F, Bandinelli S, Bartali B, Taub DD, Guralnik JM, Longo DL: The origin of age-related proinflammatory state. Blood 2005; 105(6):2294–2229.
7. Balducci L, Hardy CL, Lyman GH: Hemopoiesis and aging. Cancer Treat Res 2005;124:109–131.
8. Ershler WB, Sheng S, McKelvey J, Artz AS, Denduluri N, Tecson J, Taub DD, Brant LJ, Ferrucci L, Longo DL: Serum erythropoietin and aging: a longitudinal analysis. J Am Ger Soc 2005;53:1360–1365.
9. Ferrucci L, Guralnik L, Woodman RC, Bandinelli S, Lauretani F, Corsi AM, Chaves PH, Ershler WB, Longo DL. Proinflammatory state and circulating erythropoietin in persons with and without anemia. Am J Med 2005;118(11):1288.

10. Duthie et al, in Balducci L; Lyman GH; Ershler WB; Extermann M: Comprehensive Geriatric Oncology 2nd edition, Taylor & Francis, London, 2004.

11. Baraldi-Junkins CA, Beck AC, Rothstein G: Hematopoiesis and cytokines. Relevance to cancer and aging. Hematol Oncol Clin North Am 2000;14(1):45.

12. Ganz T: Iron metabolism and age. In: Balducci L, Ershler WB, Degaetano G. Blood disorders in the elderly. Cambridge University Press, in press.

13. Auerbach M, Ballard H, Trout JR, et al.: Intravenous iron optimizes the response to recombinant human erythropoietin in cancer patients with chemotherapy-related anemia.: A multicenter, open-label, randomized trial. J Clin Oncol 2004;22:1301–1307.

14. CardenasVM, Mulla ZD, Ortiz M, Graham DV: Iron deficiency and *Helicobacter pylori* infection in the United States. Am J Epidemiol 2006;163(2):127–134.

15. Norman EJ, Morrison JA: Screening elderly populations for cobalamin (vitamin B12) deficiency using the urinary methylmalonic acid assay by gas chromatography mass spectrometry. Am J Med 1993;94(6):589–594.

16. Solomon AL: Disorders of cobalamin (Vitamin B12) metabolism: Emerging concepts in pathophysiology, diagnosis and treatment. Blood Rev 2006;Jun 29.

17. Sipponen P, Laxen F, Huotari K, et al.: Prevalence of low vitamin B12 and high homocysteine in serum of an elderly male population: association with atrophic gastritis and *Helicobacter pylori.* Infect Scand J Gastroenterol 2003;38:1209–1216.

18. Slhub J, Jacques PF, Roenberg IH, et al.: Serum total homocysteine concentrations in the third National Health and nutrition Examination Survey (1991–1994): population references ranges and contribution of vitamin status to high serum concentrations. Ann Intern Med 1999;131:331–339.

19. Rampersaud GC, Kowell GP, Bailey LC: Folate: a key to optimizing health and reducing disease risk in the elderly. J Am Coll Nutr 2003;22(1):1–8.

20. Pelucchi C, Talamini R, Negri E: Folate intake and risk of oral and pharyngeal cancer. Ann Oncol 2003;14(11):1677–1681.

21. Makoni SN, Laber DA: Clinical spectrum of Myelophthisis in cancer patients. Am J Hematol 2004;76:92–93.

22. Karakelides H, Sreekumaran NK: Sarcopenia of aging and its metabolic impact. Curr Top Dev Biol 2005;68:123–148.

23. Walston A, Headley EC, Ferrucci L, et al.: Research agenda for frailty in older adults: toward a better understanding of physiology and etiology. Summary from the American Geriatrics Society/National Institute on Aging Research Conference on Frailty in Older Adults. J Am Geriatr Soc 2006;54(6):991–1001.

24. Curt GA, Breitbart W, Cella D, Groopman JE, Horning SJ, Itri LM, Johnson DH, Miaskowski C, Scherr SL, Portenoy RK, Vogelzang NJ: Impact of cancer-related fatigue on the lives of patients: new findings from the fatigue coalition. Oncologist 2000;5(5):353–360.

25. Penninx BW, Pahor M, Cesari M, et al.: Anemia is associated with disability and decreased physical performance and muscle strength in the elderly. J Am Geriatr Soc 2004;52:719–724.

26. Penninx BW, Guralnik JM, Onder G, et al.: Anemia and decline in physical performance among older persons. Am J Med, 2003;115:104–110.

27. Cesari M, Penninx BW, Lauretani F, et al.: Hemoglobin levels and skeletal muscle: results from the INCHIANTI study. J Gerontol A Biol Med Sci 2004;59:238–241.

28. Chaves PH, Sumba RD, Leng SX, Woodman RC, Ferrucci L, Guralnik JM, Fried LP: Impact of anemia and cardiovascular diseases on frailty status of community dwelling women. The Women Health and Aging Studies I and II. J Gerontol A Biol Sci Med Sci 2005;60:729–735.

29. Chaves PH, Xue QL, Guralnik JM, Ferrucii L, Volpato S, Fried LP: What constitutes normal hemoglobin concentration in community dwelling disabled older women? J Am Ger Soc 2004;52(11):1811–1816.

30. Tralongo P, Respini D, Ferrau F: Fatigue and aging. Crit Rev Oncol Hematol 2003;48(Suppl):S57–S64.

31. Extermann M, Chen A, Cantor AB, Corcoran MB, Meyer J, Grendys E, Cavanaugh D, Antonek S, Camarata A, Haley WE, Balducci L: Predictors of tolerance from chemotherapy in older patients: a prospective pilot study. Eur J Cancer 2002;38(11): 1466–1473.

32. Schrijvers D, Highley M, DeBruyn E, Van Oosterom AT, Vermorken JB: Role of red blood cell in pharmacokinetics of chemotherapeutic agents. Anticancer Drugs 1999;10:147–153.

33. Ratain MJ, Schilsky RL, Choi KE, et al.: Adaptive control of etoposide administration: impact of interpatient pharmacodynamic variability. Clin Pharmacol Ther 1989;45:226–233.

34. Silber JH, Fridman M, Di Paola RS, et al.: First-cycle Blood counts and subsequent neutropenia, dose reduction or delay in early stage breast cancer therapy. J Clin Oncol 1998;16:2392–2400.

35. Wolff D, Culakova E, Poniewierski MS, et al.: Predictors of chemotherapy-induced neutropenia and its complications: results from a propsective nationwide registry. J Support Oncol 2005;3(6 Suppl 4):24–25.

36. Pickett JL, Theberge DC, Brown WS, Schweitzer SU, Nissenson AR: Normalizing hematocrit in dialysis patients improves brain function. Am J Kidney Dis 1999;33(6):1122–1130.

37. Zamboni V, Cesari M, Zuccala G, et al.: Anemia and cognitive performance in hospitalized older patients: results from the GIFA study. Int J Geriatr Psychiatry 2006;21: 529–534.

38. Chaves PH, Carlson MC, Ferrucci L, et al.: Association between mild anemia and executive function impairment in community dwelling older women: the women health and aging study II. J Am Geriatr Soc 2006;54:1429–1435.

39. Atti AR, Palmer K, Volpato S, et al.: Anemia increases the risk of dementia in cognitively intact elderly. Neurobiol Aging 2006;27:278–284.

40. Donovan KA, Small BJ, Andrykowski MA, et al.: Cognitive functioning after adjuvant chemotherapy and/or radiotherapy for early stage breast carcinoma. Cancer 2005;104:2499–2507.

41. Sazama K, DeChristopher PJ, Dodd R, Harrison CR, et al.: Practice parameter for the recognition, management and prevention of adverse consequences of blood transfusion. Arch Pathol Lab Med 2000;124:61–70.

42. Heiss MM, Mempel W, Delanoff C, Jauch KW, Gabka C, Mempel M, Dieterich HJ, Eissner HJ, Schildberg FW: Blood transfusion-modulated tumor recurrence: first results of a randomized study of autologous versus allogeneic blood transfusion in colorectal cancer surgery. J Clin Oncol 1994;12(9):1859–1867.

43. Schiffer CA: Diagnosis and management of refractoriness to platelet transfusion. Blood Rev 2001;15(4):175–180.

44. Kikuchi M, Inagaki T, Shinagawa N: Five-year survival of older people with anemia: variation with hemoglobin concentration. J Am Geriatr Soc 2001;49:1226–1228.

45. Izaks GJ, Westendorp RGJ, Knook DL: The definition of anemia in older persons. JAMA 1999;281(18):1714–1719.

46. Penninx BW, Pahor M, Woodman RC, et al.: Anemia in old age is associated with increased mortality and hospitalization. J Gerontol Med Sci 2006;61:474–479.

47. Zakai NA, Katz R, Hirsch C, et al.: A prospective study of anemia status, hemoglobin concentration, and mortality in an elderly cohort: the Cardiovasccular Health Study. Arch Intern Med 2005;165:2214–2220.
48. Culleton BF, Manns BJ, Zhang J, et al.: Impact of anemia on hospitalization and mortality in older adults. Blood 2006;15(107):3841–3846.
49. Anía BJ, Suman VJ, Fairbanks VF, Rademacher DM, Melton LJ, 3rd: Incidence of anemia in older people: an epidemiologic study in a well defined population. J Am Geriatr Soc 1997;45:825–831.
50. Osterborg A: New erythropoietic proteins: rationale and clinical data. Semin Oncol 2004;31(3 Suppl 8):12–18.
51. Canon J-L, Vansteenkiste J, Bodoky G, et al.: Final results of a randomized, double-blind, active-controlled trial of darbepoetin alfa administered once every 3 weeks (Q#W) for the treatment of anemia in patients receiving multicycle chemotherapy. Am Soc Clin Oncol Proc, 2005;23:16S LBA8284.
52. McDougall JC: CERA (Continuous Erythropoietin Receptor Activator): a new erythropoiesis stimulating agent for the treatment of anemia. Curr Hematol Rep 2005;4:436–440.
53. Stead RG, Lambert J, Wessels D, et al.: Evaluation of the safety and pharmacodynamics of Hematide, a novel erythropoietic agent, in a phase 1, double-blind, placebo-controlled, dose-escalation study in healthy volunteers. Blood 2006;108(6):1830–1834.
54. Glaspy J, Bukowski R, Steinberg C, et al.: Impact of therapy with epoetin alfa on clinical outcomes in patients with non-myeloid malignancies during cancer chemotherapy in community oncology practices. J Clin Oncol 1997;5:1218–1234.
55. Demetri GD, Kris M, Wade J, et al.: Quality of life benefits in chemotherapy patients treated with epoetin alfa is independent from disease response and tumor type. Result of a prospective community oncology study. The procrit study group. J Clin Oncol 1998;16:3412–3420.
56. Gabrilove JL, Einhorn LH, Livingston RB, et al.: Once weekly dosing of epoetin alfa is similar to three-times weekly dosing in increasing hemoglobin and quality of life. Proc Am Soc Clin Oncol 1999;18:574A.
57. Littlewood TJ, Bajetta E, Nortier JW, et al. Effects of epoetin alfa on hematologic parameters and quality of life in cancer patients receiving nonplatinum chemotherapy: results of a randomized, double-blind, placebo-controlled trial. J Clin Oncol 2001;19(11):2865–2874.
58. Bohlius J, Langersiepen S, Schwarzer G, et al.: Recombinant human erythropoietins and cancer patients: updated meta-analysis of 57 studies including 9353 patients. J Natl Cancer Inst 2006;98(10):708–714.
59. Hayman JA, Langa KM, Kabeto MU, et al.: Estimating the cost of informal caregiving for elderly patients with cancer. J Clin Oncol 2001;19:3219–3225.
60. Bennett CL, Luminari S, Nissenson AR, et al.: Pure red cell aplasia and epoetin therapy. N Engl J Med 2004;351:1403–1408.
61. Henke M, Laszig R, Rube C, et al. Erythropoietin to treat head and neck cancer in patients with anaemia undergoing radiotherapy: randomized, double-blind, placebo-controlled trial. Lancet 2003;362:1255–1260.
62. Leyland-Jones B. Breast cancer trial with erythropoietin terminated unexpectedly. Lancet Oncol 2003;4:459–469.
63. Henke M, Mattern D, Pepe M, et al.: Do erythropoietin receptors on cancer cells explain unexpected clinical findings? J Clin Oncol 2006;24(29):4708–4713.

64. Rizzo JD, Lichtin AE, Woolf SH, et al.: Use of epoetin in patients with cancer: evidence-based clinical practice guidelines of the American Society of Clinical Oncology and the American Society of Hematology. J Clin Oncol 2002;20:4083–4107.
65. Henry DH, Gordan LN, Charu V, et al.: Randomized, open-label comparison of epoetin alfa extended dosing (80 000 U Q2W) vs weekly dosing (40 000 U QW) in patients with chemotherapy-induced anemia. Curr Med Res Opin 2006;22(7):1403–1413.
66. Cremieux PY, Finkelstein SN, Berndt ER, Crawford J, Slavin MB: Cost effectiveness, quality-adjusted life-years and supportive care. Recombinant human erythropoietin as a treatment of cancer-associated anaemia. Pharmacoeconomics 1999;16(5 Pt 1):459–472.
67. Anonymous: Integrating Economic Analysis Into Cancer Clinical Trials: The National Cancer Institute-American Society of Clinical Oncology Economics Workbook. J Natl Cancer Inst Monograph, 1998;24:1–28.

Chapter 9

Erythropoietin Deficiency and Late-Life Anemia

Bindu Kanapuru, Andrew S. Artz, and William B. Ershler

Introduction

As discussed extensively in this volume, anemia occurs with increasing frequency as people age. Curiously, a specific explanation for anemia is less readily apparent for older patients and approximately one-third of those with anemia over 65 years of age meet criteria for "Unexplained Anemia" (UA) as defined by Guralnik (1) and Artz (2). Although, by definition, those with kidney disease have an explanation for anemia and would not be considered to have UA, erythropoietin (EPO) insufficiency independent of overt renal excretory failure may be one component of this disorder. Certainly, other factors, including the coexistence of occult inflammatory disease, age-associated cytokine dysregulation (independent of inflammation) and androgen deficiency are also likely to contribute. In this chapter, EPO insufficiency will be considered in the context of anemia in general, and late-life UA in particular.

Erythropoietin

EPO, a glycoprotein secreted by interstitial cells in the kidney (3), has a major role in regulating erythropoiesis in humans. EPO is primarily regulated by blood oxygen content and secretion is stimulated by hypoxia (4, 5). EPO stimulates hematopoiesis by increasing proliferation (6) and preventing apoptosis (3, 7) of erythroid progenitor cells. The primary site of action of EPO in the bone marrow is the late stage colony-forming unit erythroid (CFU-E). EPO induces these cells to both proliferate and mature as well as to become resistant to apoptosis (3, 7).

Erythropoietin and Aging

Under normal conditions (i.e., without disease) erythropoietin serum levels increase with advancing age. In this regard, the data from cross-sectional studies are both limited and conflicting (8–14), but that from longitudinal study is quite revealing. For example, samples obtained from the National Institute on Aging (NIA) Baltimore Longitudinal Study of Aging (BLSA) clearly demonstrated a gradual and sustained rise in serum EPO among healthy individuals as they age (Fig. 9.1) (15). Importantly, for those in the BLSA analysis who were to develop hypertension and/or diabetes during their tenure as study participants, the slope of the incline was significantly less pronounced (Fig. 9.2). Thus, it was speculated that renal erythropoietin production or secretion was negatively influenced by the same disease processes that impair renal excretory function (i.e., diabetes and hypertension). While there is evidence that erythropoietin serum levels tend to increase with advancing age, for some the rise is of insufficient magnitude to maintain a hemoglobin concentration in the normal range (2). This observation has also been reported for patients with diabetes, even without associated measurable renal insufficiency (16).

Erythropoietin Insufficiency in Renal Failure

The prevalence of anemia increases incrementally with declines in creatinine clearance (17, 18). This has been attributed to several mechanisms including: (1) decreased capacity for EPO production or secretion;

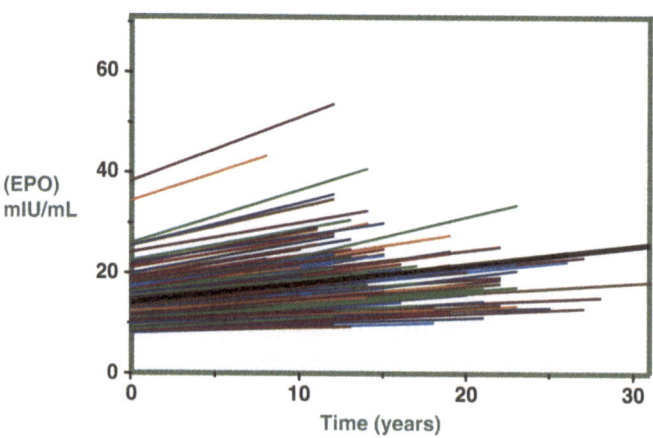

Fig. 9.1. Serum erythropoietin levels over time in normal adults. Erythropoietin levels measured at two year intervals for a minimum of four determinations, each separated by two years. Each of the thin lines indicates the predicted erythropoietin level for each individual. The bold line represents the population average change over time (15)

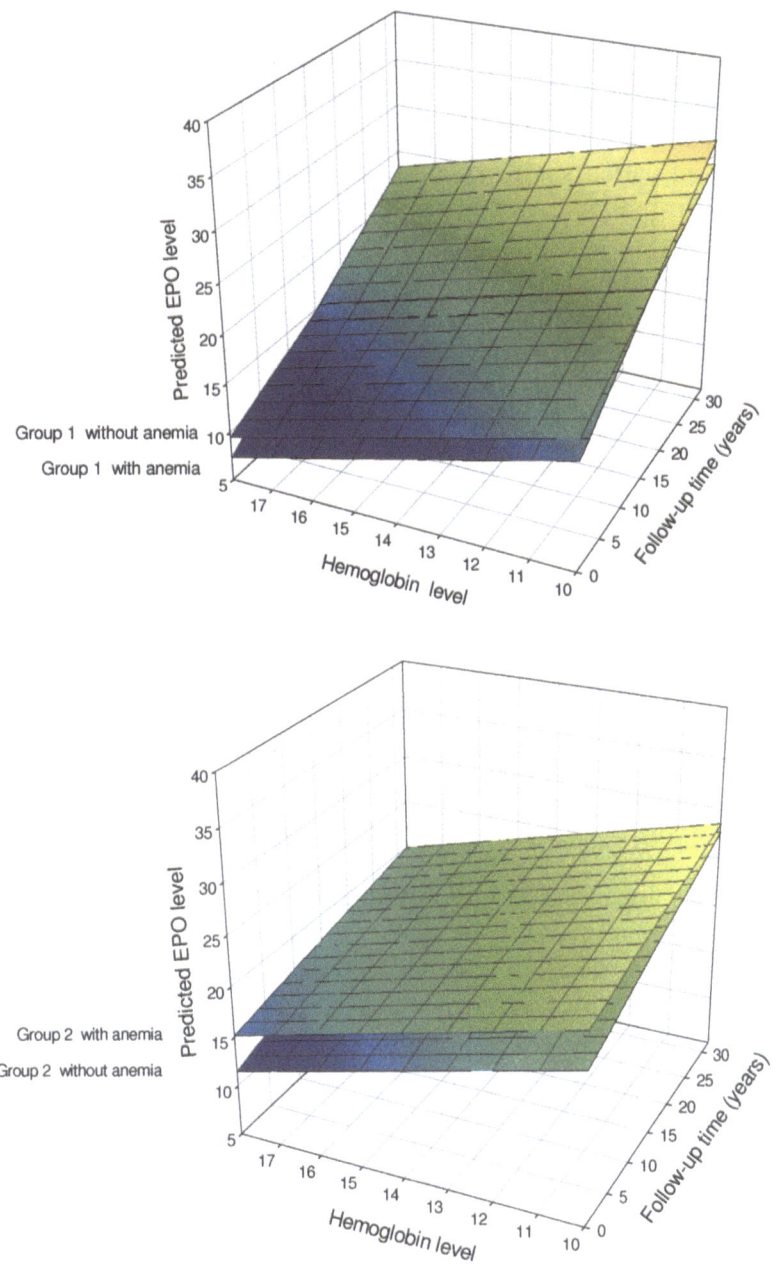

Fig. 9.2. Predicted erythropoietin levels using a linear mixed-effects model as a function of hemoglobin level (g/dL) and time (years). The top panel projects results for those who remained healthy free of hypertension or diabetes (Group 1, $n = 84$), some of whom, however, developed anemia ($n = 15$), whereas the remainder did not ($n = 69$). The bottom panel projects results for those individuals who during the course of their participation on this study developed diabetes, hypertension, or both conditions ($n = 59$). Some of these individuals developed anemia ($n = 15$), whereas others did not ($n = 44$) From Ershler et al. (15)

(2) inadequate bone marrow response to EPO; and, (3) presence of EPO inhibitors (19). Most currently agree the predominant mechanism is EPO deficiency (20, 21). It has been recognized for several decades that EPO levels were low in anemic hemodialysis patients (22, 23). Additionally, work by Zucker and colleagues demonstrated decreased EPO levels in patients with anemia and renal failure but no measurable inhibitors or inadequate marrow response to exogenous EPO when anemic kidney failure patients were compared with iron deficiency or nonanemic individuals (24). Furthermore, in a sheep model of chronic kidney failure and uremia, excellent erythropoietic response and correction of anemia was observed by treatment with erythropoietin-rich plasma (25). More recently, epidemiological data capitalizing on the development of more sensitive serum EPO assays have further clarified the tight negative correlation of EPO and kidney function. For example, the InChianti Study, a prospective population based analysis of 436 men and 569 women (65 years or older), found that low-hemoglobin levels and lower erythropoietin levels were clearly demonstrable in people with creatinine clearance of 30 mL/min and below (26). Finally EPO replacement has been shown to correct anemia in almost all iron-replete anemia patients with CKD (27). These data, and much more indicate the importance of EPO deficiency in pathogenesis of anemia associated with kidney failure.

Erythropoietin Response in Patients with Iron Deficiency

EPO levels are usually higher in anemic patients with iron deficiency than when anemia is caused by other processes, such as inflammation or renal insufficiency (28–31). Pregnant rats fed with an iron-deficient diet were found to have significantly increased EPO levels (32) and, similarly elevated levels were found in iron-deficient pregnant women (33). Serum EPO levels in rheumatoid arthritis (RA) patients with coexisting iron deficiency and anemia were higher than those with RA and anemia but normal iron stores (34). Thus, to the extent that iron deficiency contributes to anemia, one would expect to observe appropriately elevated EPO levels. And, as a corollary, if such is not observed, contributing factors, such as inflammation or renal insufficiency should be considered. Similarly, EPO levels in iron-deficient elderly anemic patients, although higher than those without iron deficiency, were found to be lower than expected for the degree of anemia by several investigators (2, 10, 11, 13). Thus, we speculate that even for those elderly patients with iron deficiency, the late-life factors that, in composite, result in UA (discussed below) are also contributing to the observed anemia.

Erythropoietin Insufficiency in HIV Anemia

Anemia is an extremely common finding in patients infected with human immunodeficiency virus (HIV). For example, Sullivan and colleagues reported a 1-year incidence of anemia as 37% among patients with clinical AIDS, 12% among patients with CD4+ cell count <200 cells/mm^3 in the absence of an AIDS-defining clinical condition, and 3% among HIV-infected individuals with neither clinical nor immunologic AIDS (35). This was particularly remarkable because the criterion for 'anemia' in this survey was a hemoglobin level below 10 g/dL. With HIV infection, the cause of anemia is considered multifactorial and may involve direct bone marrow toxicity by the virus, nutrient deficiencies, and the myelosuppressive effects of certain antiviral drugs (36, 37). Low levels of EPO have been demonstrated consistently in HIV patients and these correlate significantly with the presence of anemia. The adequacy of endogenous EPO response in anemic HIV patients was assessed in 42 subjects and compared to the response observed in patients with anemia of chronic disease or iron deficiency. With comparable degrees of anemia, EPO levels in AIDS patients and those with chronic disease were lower than those with iron deficiency (31). Similar results were also reported by Spivak and colleagues who demonstrated the mean incremental increase in serum immunoreactive EPO levels for a given decline in hemoglobin was significantly less in AIDS patients when compared to those with iron deficiency (38, 39). It is also notable that the use of recombinant human EPO to treat anemia in HIV infected patients, particularly those with low-EPO levels, has been shown to correct anemia and improve quality of life (40, 41).

Erythropoietin Deficiency in Diabetes Mellitus

Anemia is a common complication of both type I and II diabetes mellitus. In a cross sectional survey of 820 patients with diabetes in long-term follow up, the prevalence of anemia defined as a hemoglobin concentration of <12 g/dL in women and <13 g/dL in men was two to three times greater in diabetic patients with comparable renal impairment and iron stores, as observed in the general population (42). Anemia occurs in patients with only minor derangement of renal excretory function and at any level of glomerular filtration. Furthermore, anemia is generally more severe in diabetic patients than nondiabetics (43, 44). The pathogenesis of anemia in diabetes has been attributed predominantly to reduced levels of EPO (42, 45, 46). In a study conducted by Bosman et al., serum EPO levels in anemic diabetic patients failed to increase and were much lower than the levels in nondiabetic anemic patients and in patients with microcytic anemia (44). In a cross-sectional study of 604 diabetic patients, more than 71% of those with anemia demonstrated functional EPO deficiency and this was independent of the severity of renal impairment (46). Similar results were also reported in type I diabetic patients without overt nephropathy by Cotroneo et al. (47) and Thomas et al. (45). In patients with normal serum creatinine, EPO level was predictive of a more rapid deterioration of renal function (43).

Numerous mechanisms have been proposed to explain the low EPO levels in diabetic patients including presence of structural renal abnormalities and a possible inhibitory effect of advanced glycosylation end products on EPO production (48). Curiously, the presence of anemia in patients with DM has been associated with neuropathy (47, 49, 50) and it has even been proposed that reduced EPO levels are causally related to diabetic autonomic polyneuropathy (51) with efferent sympathetic denervation (44, 52). Regardless of the mechanism, EPO insufficiency is an important cause of anemia in patients with diabetes and studies are underway to assess the value of treatment with recombinant EPO in terms of quality of life, physical function and the progression of diabetic complications.

The Role of EPO Deficiency in the Late-Life Occurrence of UA

Investigation into the etiology of anemia in individuals older than 65 years of age revealed a high percentage of cases (15–45%) where no cause was definable (1, 2, 9). Currently termed "Unexplained Anemia," the likelihood is that this condition is the result of not one, but several contributing factors which, in composite, result in the anemic condition. Several of these factors are listed in Table 9.1 and discussed in the paragraphs below.

Kidney Function and Aging. Of the many physiological changes that occur with age, there is a gradual decline in renal excretory function (53). In the absence of disease, however, renal production of EPO appears adequate even with the added demands of diminished stem cell proliferative capacity necessitating compensatory levels as evident by the continued rise in serum EPO with age in healthy subjects (15). However, it is possible that this reserve in EPO production capacity runs out in very late-life, or earlier in patients with renal damage secondary to diabetes, hypertension or other disease processes. Thus, it is likely that renal insufficiency, either on the basis of age alone, or in combination with underlying disease contributes to UA by its associated decline in EPO production.

Inflammation and Age-Associated Cytokine Dysregulation. In most elderly, particularly frail elderly, there exist at least one, and frequently several comorbid conditions which have, at their root, inflammation. One common

Table 9.1. Factors contributing to unexplained anemia in the elderly

Factor	Mechanism	EPO deficiency involved?
Renal insufficiency	Certain age-associated diseases including diabetes and hypertension impaired kidney function. Also, aging itself is associated with a gradual decline in GFR.	Directly
Inflammation	Cytokine-induced hepcidin inhibits iron absorption and mobilization. Cytokines may also inhibit EPO synthesis or ligand-binding.	Indirectly and directly
Age-associated cytokine dysregulation	As above (Inflammation)	Indirectly and directly
Stem cell	Regenerative capacity diminished	Indirectly
Myelodysplasia	Stem cell proliferative impairment	Indirectly
Androgen deficiency	Age-associated decline	Indirectly

feature of chronic inflammatory disease is anemia and to the extent that underlying inflammatory disease is unrecognized, coexisting anemia might be miscategorized as UA. Artz and colleagues (2) recognized this and in their nursing home series of UA patients (mentioned above), excluded from analysis those with an elevated erythrocyte sedimentation rate (ESR) or C-reactive protein (CRP). However, even with this screen, it is likely undiagnosed inflammatory processes contribute to some extent to the composite picture of UA. Compounding this, it is now generally accepted that the serum levels of certain proinflammatory cytokines rise with age, even in the absence of inflammatory disease. For example, interleukin-6, now considered a biochemical marker of frailty, is typically measurable only in sub-picogram quantities in the absence of acute inflammation in young adults but rises gradually after menopause (or andropause) and its level correlates with several features of the frail phenotype, including sarcopenia, osteopenia, functional decline, and anemia (54–62). Thus, to the extent that cytokine dysregulation occurs with advancing age, even in the absence of overt inflammatory disease, these same cytokines may contribute to the development of anemia. It is noteworthy that the cytokine most frequently associated with aging and frailty, IL-6, is also the one most commonly associated with inflammation-associated hepcidin upregulation, reduced iron availability, and anemia (63–66).

Stem Cells and Aging. Studies conducted in mice demonstrated reduced proliferative capacity of erythroid progenitor cells with age (67, 68). However, even with this decline, old mice do not become anemic; suggesting in the absence of disease, the acquired intrinsic stem cell defect is compensated by an increase in other factors, including an increase in erythropoietin level. In fact, this may explain the aforementioned rise in serum EPO observed in the BLSA study (15). However, if there is impairment in EPO production, such as in advanced age or with kidney disease, diabetes or inflammatory disease (as described above), insufficiently compensated augmentation of the age-associated decline in stem cell proliferative capacity may be an important component of the pathogenesis of UA.

Myelodysplasia and UA. Myelodysplasia (MDS) occurs with increasing frequency in late-life (69). Although it usually can be diagnosed on the peripheral blood smear by dysplastic white blood cell features associated with macrocytic erythrocytes, it may present as anemia alone, particularly in the elderly (70). Examination of a bone marrow aspirate and biopsy provide more diagnostic accuracy, but if the anemia is mild, this may not be clinically warranted outside a research setting. Thus, some patients considered to have UA may actually have MDS although it is likely this would comprise a small fraction of the total UA pool.

Circulating EPO levels in myelodysplastic syndromes are typically elevated (71, 72) likely representing a compensatory effect to overcome intrinsic defects within the progenitor cell compartments. Bone marrow CFU-E and BFU-E in patients with MDS grew poorly in vitro despite high levels of added EPO (72). The inhibited proliferative response was shown to be associated with the absence of STAT5 (Signal Transducer and Activator of Transription-5) suggesting a defect in the Epo-receptor (EpoR) signal transduction pathway contributes to anemia in myelodysplasia (73).

Androgen Deficiency and UA. Epidemiological studies have demonstrated a negative correlation between circulating androgen levels and hemoglobin concentration in an elderly population (74) raising the speculation that an age-associated decline in androgens is yet another contributing factor to UA. One mechanism that testosterone enhances erythropoiesis is by enhancing renal EPO secretion (75). In older, compared with younger rats, orchiectomy reduced EPO release from kidney cells in response to hypoxia to much greater extent. Furthermore, replacement of testosterone restored the production of EPO to normal levels indicating that in aging rats hypoxia induced release of EPO may be diminished by androgen deficiency (76). In anemic human subjects replacement with testosterone was shown to increase levels of EPO (77). Hence indirectly androgen deficiency could cause anemia by reducing EPO levels.

Although there remains no direct evidence that EPO levels are decreased in patients with androgen deficiency, studies have shown a synergistic action of increasing concentrations of testosterone and EPO in stimulating erythropoiesis in vitro. These effects were completely blocked by pretreatment with the androgen antagonists cyproterone and flutamide (78).

Conclusion

An inadequate erythropoietin response contributes to the pathogenesis of anemia under a variety of circumstances. It may occur as a result of underlying renal disease, age-associated renal decline, or in association with inhibitory cytokines or other factors. Unexplained anemia (UA), that fraction of all anemias that defy simple etiological classification, may be considered a composite of several different causative factors. Many of these either directly or indirectly mediate their effect by limiting erythropoietin response. To the extent that EPO deficiency contributes to UA, it is likely that treatment with recombinant erythropoietin or similar agents would raise hemoglobin very effectively. However, it remains to be demonstrated whether such treatment would be associated with improved quality of life, physical or cognitive function and whether administration could be accomplished safely in frail, elderly anemic patients.

References

1. Guralnik JM, Eisenstaedt RS, Ferrucci L, Klein HG, Woodman RC. Prevalence of anemia in persons 65 years and older in the United States: evidence for a high rate of unexplained anemia. Blood 2004;104(8):2263–8.
2. Artz AS, Fergusson D, Drinka PJ, et al. Mechanisms of unexplained anemia in the nursing home. J Am Geriatr Soc 2004;52(3):423–7.
3. Fisher JW. Erythropoietin: physiology and pharmacology update. Exp Biol Med (Maywood) 2003;228(1):1–14.
4. Erslev AJ. Erythropoietin. N Engl J Med 1991;324(19):1339–44.
5. Erslev AJ. Clinical erythrokinetics: a critical review. Blood Rev 1997;11(3):160–7.
6. Yoshimura A, Arai K. Physician education: the erythropoietin receptor and signal transduction. Oncologist 1996;1(5):337–9.
7. Akimoto T, Kusano E, Inaba T, et al. Erythropoietin regulates vascular smooth muscle cell apoptosis by a phosphatidylinositol 3 kinase-dependent pathway. Kidney Int 2000;58(1):269–82.
8. Goodnough LT, Price TH, Parvin CA. The endogenous erythropoietin response and the erythropoietic response to blood loss anemia: the effects of age and gender. J Lab Clin Med 1995;126(1):57–64.

9. Joosten E, Pelemans W, Hiele M, Noyen J, Verhaeghe R, Boogaerts MA. Prevalence and causes of anaemia in a geriatric hospitalized population. Gerontology 1992; 38(1–2):111–7.

10. Kario K, Matsuo T, Kodama K, Nakao K, Asada R. Reduced erythropoietin secretion in senile anemia. Am J Hematol 1992;41(4):252–7.

11. Kario K, Matsuo T, Nakao K. Serum erythropoietin levels in the elderly. Gerontology 1991;37(6):345–8.

12. Mori M, Murai Y, Hirai M, et al. Serum erythropoietin titers in the aged. Mech Ageing Dev 1988;46(1–3):105–9.

13. Nafziger J, Pailla K, Luciani L, Andreux JP, Saint-Jean O, Casadevall N. Decreased erythropoietin responsiveness to iron deficiency anemia in the elderly. Am J Hematol 1993;43(3):172–6.

14. Powers JS, Krantz SB, Collins JC, et al. Erythropoietin response to anemia as a function of age. J Am Geriatr Soc 1991;39(1):30–2.

15. Ershler WB, Sheng S, McKelvey J, et al. Serum erythropoietin and aging: a longitudinal analysis. J Am Geriatr Soc 2005;53(8):1360–5.

16. Ahn SH, Garewal HS. Low erythropoietin level can cause anemia in patients without advanced renal failure. Am J Med 2004;116(4):280–1.

17. Astor BC, Muntner P, Levin A, Eustace JA, Coresh J. Association of kidney function with anemia: the Third National Health and Nutrition Examination Survey (1988–1994). Arch Intern Med 2002;162(12):1401–8.

18. McClellan W, Aronoff SL, Bolton WK, et al. The prevalence of anemia in patients with chronic kidney disease. Curr Med Res Opin 2004;20(9):1501–10.

19. Urabe A, Saito T, Fukamachi H, Kubota M, Takaku F. Serum erythropoietin titers in the anemia of chronic renal failure and other hematological states. Int J Cell Cloning 1987;5(3):202–8.

20. Pavlovic-Kentera V, Clemons GK, Djukanovic L, Biljanovic-Paunovic L. Erythropoietin and anemia in chronic renal failure. Exp Hematol 1987;15(7):785–9.

21. Rigatto C. Anemia, renal transplantation, and the anemia paradox. Semin Nephrol 2006;26(4):307–12.

22. Radtke HW, Erbes PM, Fassbinder W, Koch KM. The variable role of erythropoietin deficiency in the pathogenesis of dialysis anaemia. Proc Eur Dial Transplant Assoc 1977;14:177–83.

23. Radtke HW, Erbes PM, Schippers E, Koch KM. Serum erythropoietin concentration in anephric patients. Nephron 1978;22(4–6):361–5.

24. Zucker S, Lysik RM, Mohammad G. Erythropoiesis in chronic renal disease. J Lab Clin Med 1976;88(4):528–35.

25. Eschbach JW, Mladenovic J, Garcia JF, Wahl PW, Adamson JW. The anemia of chronic renal failure in sheep. response to erythropoietin-rich plasma in vivo. J Clin Invest 1984;74(2):434–41.

26. Ble A, Fink JC, Woodman RC, et al. Renal function, erythropoietin, and anemia of older persons: the InCHIANTI study. Arch Intern Med 2005;165(19):2222–7.

27. Eschbach JW, Varma A, Stivelman JC. Is it time for a paradigm shift? Is erythropoietin deficiency still the main cause of renal anaemia? Nephrol Dial Transplant 2002;17(Suppl 5):2–7.

28. Boyd HK, Lappin TR. Erythropoietin deficiency in the anaemia of chronic disorders. Eur J Haematol 1991;46(4):198–201.

29. Boyd HK, Lappin TR, Bell AL. Evidence for impaired erythropoietin response to anaemia in rheumatoid disease. Br J Rheumatol 1991;30(4):255–9.

30. Bruno CM, Neri S, Sciacca C, et al. Plasma erythropoietin levels in anaemic and non-anaemic patients with chronic liver diseases. World J Gastroenterol 2004;10(9):1353–6.

31. Camacho J, Poveda F, Zamorano AF, Valencia ME, Vazquez JJ, Arnalich F. Serum ery-thropoietin levels in anaemic patients with advanced human immunodeficiency virus infection. Br J Haematol 1992;82(3):608–14.

32. Horiguchi H, Oguma E, Kayama F. The effects of iron deficiency on estradiol-induced suppression of erythropoietin induction in rats: implications of pregnancy-related ane-mia. Blood 2005;106(1):67–74.

33. Milman N, Graudal N, Nielsen OJ, Agger AO. Serum erythropoietin during normal pregnancy: relationship to hemoglobin and iron status markers and impact of iron sup-plementation in a longitudinal, placebo-controlled study on 118 women. Int J Hematol 1997;66(2):159–68.

34. Takashina N, Kondo H, Kashiwazaki S. Suppressed serum erythropoietin response to anemia and the efficacy of recombinant erythropoietin in the anemia of rheumatoid arthritis. J Rheumatol 1990;17(7):885–7.

35. Sullivan PS, Hanson DL, Chu SY, Jones JL, Ward JW. Epidemiology of anemia in human immunodeficiency virus (HIV)-infected persons: results from the multistate adult and adolescent spectrum of HIV disease surveillance project. Blood 1998;91(1):301–8.

36. Kreuzer KA, Rockstroh JK. Pathogenesis and pathophysiology of anemia in HIV infec-tion. Ann Hematol 1997;75(5–6):179–87.

37. Moore RD. Anemia and human immunodeficiency virus disease in the era of highly active antiretroviral therapy. Semin Hematol 2000;37(4 Suppl 6):18–23.

38. Spivak JL. Serum immunoreactive erythropoietin in health and disease. J Perinat Med 1995;23(1–2):13–7.

39. Spivak JL, Barnes DC, Fuchs E, Quinn TC. Serum immunoreactive erythropoietin in HIV-infected patients. Jama 1989;261(21):3104–7.

40. Henry DH, Beall GN, Benson CA, et al. Recombinant human erythropoietin in the treatment of anemia associated with human immunodeficiency virus (HIV) infection and zidovudine therapy. Overview of four clinical trials. Ann Intern Med 1992;117(9):739–48.

41. Revicki DA, Brown RE, Henry DH, McNeill MV, Rios A, Watson T. Recombinant human erythropoietin and health-related quality of life of AIDS patients with anemia. J Acquir Immune Defic Syndr 1994;7(5):474–84.

42. Thomas MC, MacIsaac RJ, Tsalamandris C, Power D, Jerums G. Unrecognized anemia in patients with diabetes: a cross-sectional survey. Diabetes Care 2003;26(4):1164–9.

43. Ritz E, Haxsen V. Diabetic nephropathy and anaemia. Eur J Clin Invest 2005;35(Suppl 3): 66–74.

44. Bosman DR, Winkler AS, Marsden JT, Macdougall IC, Watkins PJ. Anemia with erythropoietin deficiency occurs early in diabetic nephropathy. Diabetes Care 2001;24(3):495–9.

45. Thomas MC, Cooper ME, Tsalamandris C, MacIsaac R, Jerums G. Anemia with impaired erythropoietin response in diabetic patients. Arch Intern Med 2005;165(4):466–9.

46. Thomas MC, Tsalamandris C, Macisaac R, Jerums G. Functional erythropoietin defi-ciency in patients with Type 2 diabetes and anaemia. Diabet Med 2006;23(5):502–9.

47. Cotroneo P, Maria Ricerca B, Todaro L, et al. Blunted erythropoietin response to ane-mia in patients with Type 1 diabetes. Diabetes Metab Res Rev 2000;16(3):172–6.

48. Dikow R, Schwenger V, Schomig M, Ritz E. How should we manage anaemia in patients with diabetes? Nephrol Dial Transplant 2002;17(Suppl 1):67–72.

49. Thomas S, Rampersad M. Anaemia in diabetes. Acta Diabetol 2004;41(Suppl 1):S13–7.

50. Winkler AS, Marsden J, Chaudhuri KR, Hambley H, Watkins PJ. Erythropoietin deple-tion and anaemia in diabetes mellitus. Diabet Med 1999;16(10):813–9.

51. Spallone V, Maiello MR, Kurukulasuriya N, et al. Does autonomic neuropathy play a role in erythropoietin regulation in non-proteinuric Type 2 diabetic patients? Diabet Med 2004;21(11):1174–80.

52. Beynon G. The influence of the autonomic nervous system in the control of erythropoietin secretion in the hypoxic rat. J Physiol 1977;266(2):347–60.

53. Lindeman RD. Overview: renal physiology and pathophysiology of aging. Am J Kidney Dis 1990;16(4):275–82.

54. Ershler WB. Interleukin-6: a cytokine for gerontologists. J Am Geriatr Soc 1993; 41(2):176–81.

55. Fagiolo U, Cossarizza A, Scala E, et al. Increased cytokine production in mononuclear cells of healthy elderly people. Eur J Immunol 1993;23(9):2375–8.

56. Ershler WB, Keller ET. Age-associated increased interleukin-6 gene expression, late-life diseases, and frailty. Annu Rev Med 2000;51:245–70.

57. Cohen HJ, Pieper CF, Harris T, Rao KM, Currie MS. The association of plasma IL-6 levels with functional disability in community-dwelling elderly. J Gerontol 1997;52(4):M201–8.

58. Leng S, Chaves P, Koenig K, Walston J. Serum interleukin-6 and hemoglobin as physiological correlates in the geriatric syndrome of frailty: a pilot study. J Am Geriatr Soc 2002;50(7):1268–71.

59. Forsey RJ, Thompson JM, Ernerudh J, et al. Plasma cytokine profiles in elderly humans. Mech Ageing Dev 2003;124(4):487–93.

60. Ferrucci L, Guralnik JM, Woodman RC, et al. Proinflammatory state and circulating erythropoietin in persons with and without anemia. Am J Med 2005;118(11):1288.

61. Ferrucci L, Harris TB, Guralnik JM, et al. Serum IL-6 level and the development of disability in older persons. J Am Geriatr Soc 1999;47(6):639–46.

62. Maggio M, Guralnik JM, Longo DL, Ferrucci L. Interleukin-6 in aging and chronic disease: a magnificent pathway. J Gerontol 2006;61(6):575–84.

63. Ganz T. Hepcidin, a key regulator of iron metabolism and mediator of anemia of inflammation. Blood 2003;102(3):783–8.

64. Nemeth E, Rivera S, Gabayan V, et al. IL-6 mediates hypoferremia of inflammation by inducing the synthesis of the iron regulatory hormone hepcidin. J Clin Invest 2004;113(9):1271–6.

65. Ganz T. Hepcidin – a peptide hormone at the interface of innate immunity and iron metabolism. Curr Top Microbiol Immunol 2006;306:183–98.

66. Wrighting DM, Andrews NC. Interleukin-6 induces hepcidin expression through STAT3. Blood 2006;108(9):3204–9.

67. Udupa KB, Lipschitz DA. Erythropoiesis in the aged mouse: II. Response to stimulation in vitro. J Lab Clin Med 1984;103(4):581–8.

68. Udupa KB, Lipschitz DA. Erythropoiesis in the aged mouse: I. Response to stimulation in vivo. J Lab Clin Med 1984;103(4):574–80.

69. Bennett JM, Kouides PA, Forman SJ. The myelodysplastic syndromes: morphology, risk assessment, and clinical management (2002). Int J Hematol 2002;76(Suppl 2):228–38.

70. Dewulf G, Gouin I, Pautas E, et al. Myelodisplasic syndromes diagnosed in a geriatric hospital: morphological profile in 100 patients. Ann Biol Clin (Paris) 2004;62(2):197–202.

71. Jacobs A, Janowska-Wieczorek A, Caro J, Bowen DT, Lewis T. Circulating erythropoietin in patients with myelodysplastic syndromes. Br J Haematol 1989;73(1):36–9.

72. Merchav S, Nielsen OJ, Rosenbaum H, et al. In vitro studies of erythropoietin-dependent regulation of erythropoiesis in myelodysplastic syndromes. Leukemia 1990;4(11):771–4.

73. Hoefsloot LH, van Amelsvoort MP, Broeders LC, et al. Erythropoietin-induced activation of STAT5 is impaired in the myelodysplastic syndrome. Blood 1997;89(5):1690–700.
74. Ferrucci L, Maggio M, Bandinelli S, et al. Low testosterone levels and the risk of anemia in older men and women. Arch Intern Med 2006;166(13):1380–8.
75. Malgor LA, Fisher JW. Effects of erythropoietin and testosterone on erythropoiesis in bone marrow of isolated perfused hind limbs of dogs. Acta Haematol 1970;43(6):321–8.
76. Wang RY, Tsai SC, Lu CC, et al. Effect of aging on erythropoietin secretion in male rats. J Gerontol 1996;51(6):B434–8.
77. Rishpon-Meyerstein N, Kilbridge T, Simone J, Fried W. The effect of testosterone on erythropoietin levels in anemic patients. Blood 1968;31(4):453–60.
78. Malgor LA, Valsecia M, Verges E, De Markowsky EE. Blockade of the in vitro effects of testosterone and erythropoietin on Cfu-E and Bfu-E proliferation by pretreatment of the donor rats with cyproterone and flutamide. Acta Physiol Pharmacol Ther Latinoam 1998;48(2):99–105.

Chapter 10

Anemia and Physical Health Decline in Old Age

Brenda WJH Penninx

In a previous chapter, it has been shown that anemia is prevalent among older persons. This chapter will describe that anemia is not only prevalent, but also has important adverse clinical consequences. For instance, anemia has been associated with decreased physical function, elevated risks for falls and fractures, cognitive impairment, and increased mortality. Notably, these detrimental effects are observed not only in elderly individuals with severe reductions in Hb, but also in those with mild anemia or low-normal Hb levels. The chapter starts with describing why good physical function is an essential clinical geriatric outcome. Subsequent sections provide research findings that have linked anemia with poor physical function and other important related outcomes. The last section summarizes the most important findings and will discuss implications for health care and future research.

Physical Function – An Important Geriatric Concept

Especially in old age, an individual often has multiple chronic conditions which may vary in severity. This is why especially in old age the full picture of the link between anemia and physical health cannot be portrayed by looking at just individual chronic diseases. Although individual diseases are important, and our system of modern medicine is often oriented toward the diagnosis and treatment of specific diseases, the consequences of single and multiple diseases can be understood best by an evaluation of the functional status of the patient. This is why, to date, a functional assessment forms the hallmark of geriatric medicine and research.

Various assessments and concepts for functional status have been proposed and used over the last two decades. These various concepts generally fit into a conceptual model, called the disablement process (1), which uses

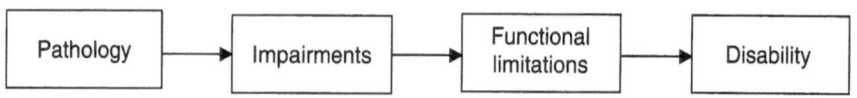

Fig. 10.1 Graphical presentation of the disablement process

concepts of the International Classification of Functioning, Disability and Health (ICF) provided by the World Health Organization (2). The disablement process model describes a pathway leading from pathology to impairment to functional limitations, and ultimately to disability (see Fig. 10.1). In this model, pathology refers to biochemical and physiological abnormalities that are detected and medically labeled as disease, injury, or as congenital or developmental conditions. Physical impairments are dysfunctions and structural abnormalities in specific body systems, such as, for instance, conceptualized in poor muscle strength, poor balance, or low walking speed. Functional limitations are experienced restrictions in performing fundamental physical actions used in daily life. Examples of functional limitations are the report of experiencing a lot of difficulty or inability with walking 1/4 mile, climbing stairs, or lifting 10 pounds, which all can be considered to be the building blocks of activities of daily life. Disability, the final stage of the disablement process, reflects how an individual's limitations interact with the demands of the environment. It indicates a restriction in or lack of ability to perform activities related to interpersonal relationships, work or school, or physical activities. For the latter, also termed physical disability, various types can be distinguished, ranging in severity. Difficulty with essential activities of daily living (ADLs) such as eating, bathing, dressing, and transferring from bed to chair indicates severe disability which usually identifies those individuals who require extensive (institutional) help. Instrumental activities of daily living (IADLs) such as housekeeping tasks, paying bills, or grocery shopping are tasks that physically and cognitively are somewhat more complicated and difficult than self-care tasks but are also necessary for independent living.

The number of older persons living with physical disability increases dramatically with increasing age. Data from the US National Health Interview Survey of Disability show that of the women aged 65 years and older, 18.8% needs help with (instrumental) activities of daily living at home, which is 10.9% in men (3). At the age of 85 years or older, 54.8% of the women and 36.9% of the men are needing help with (instrumental) activities of daily living. One of the key paradoxes in gerontology is that although women live longer than men, they live with more physical disability at older age. This is for a large part caused by the fact that the prevalence of nonlethal but disabling chronic diseases is generally higher in older women than in older men.

Physical disability status has been demonstrated in epidemiological studies to be one of the most potent of all health status indicators in predicting adverse outcomes such as mortality, hospitalization, and nursing home admission (4–6). This is because disability measures are able to capture the impact of the presence and severity of multiple pathologies, including physical, cognitive, and psychological conditions, and the potential synergistic effects of these conditions on overall health status. In line with this, older adults themselves report that they worry about their risk of disability, often more than about disease itself, because function decline changes the scope of their daily life and threatens their ability to live independently. Since the adverse impact of disability on outcomes such as hospitalization, health care utilization, and nursing home admission is large, it is not surprising that physical disability has been associated with largely increased health care costs. In a US study among 843 persons 72 years or older, those with ADL disability were found to spend 10,000 USD more on 2-year costs for hospital, outpatient, nursing home, and home care services than those without ADL disability (7).

Anemia Associated with Physical Decline

There are now several lines of evidence illustrating that anemia is a significant predictor of physical decline and disability in older adults. The effect of anemia on mobility in elderly women has been assessed in two longitudinal population-based studies, the Women's Health and Aging Studies (WHAS) I and II that evaluated the onset and progression of disability in community-dwelling elderly women (8). In these studies, the relationship between anemia and subsequent progression of disability was studied in a subgroup of 633 women, aged 70–80 years old. Mobility was assessed as either self-reported difficulty in walking 1/4 mile or climbing 10 steps, or objectively with the Short Physical Performance Battery (SPPB), a series of tests consisting of an assessment of standing balance, a timed walk, and a timed test of five chair rises, which primarily test lower extremity function. The SPPB has been shown to be both reliable and sensitive to change and to be highly predictive of subsequent disability, nursing home admission, reduced independence, and hospitalization (9–11).

The results indicated that the progression of mobility difficulty was lowest at a Hb concentration of 14 g/dL and increased continuously as Hb concentration declined below this value (8). At an Hb level below 12 g/dL the prevalence of mobility difficulty was twice that seen at 14 g/dL. Adjustment for disease, physical impairment, demographic factors, and other health indicators commonly associated with decline of physical function did not substantially change the results of the study. The authors concluded that the risk of mobility difficulty is not constant within the range of WHO-defined "normal" Hb concentrations (12–16 g/dL), but rather increases continuously over a range of Hb concentrations that would be considered low-normal by current standards (41). These authors interpreted their results to suggest that an Hb concentration of 12 g/dL may be an inappropriate criterion for defining anemia in older women, and that physiological consequences rather than statistical distribution may be a more clinically meaningful way to define the Hb threshold for anemia.

The effects of anemia on physical performance have also been assessed in another recent study of the EPESE cohort (12). In that study, plasma Hb concentration of 1,146 subjects (mean age 77 ± 5 years; 70% female) was measured and physical performance was assessed with the SPPB at baseline and 4 years later. After correction for baseline performance score, health status, and demographic characteristics, physical performance declined more over 4 years in subjects with WHO-defined anemia than in nonanemic subjects. The association of anemia with impairment of physical performance was seen in both men and women (Fig. 10.2). The physical decline in women with borderline anemia (Hb concentration = 12–13 g/dL) was significantly greater than in those subjects with Hb

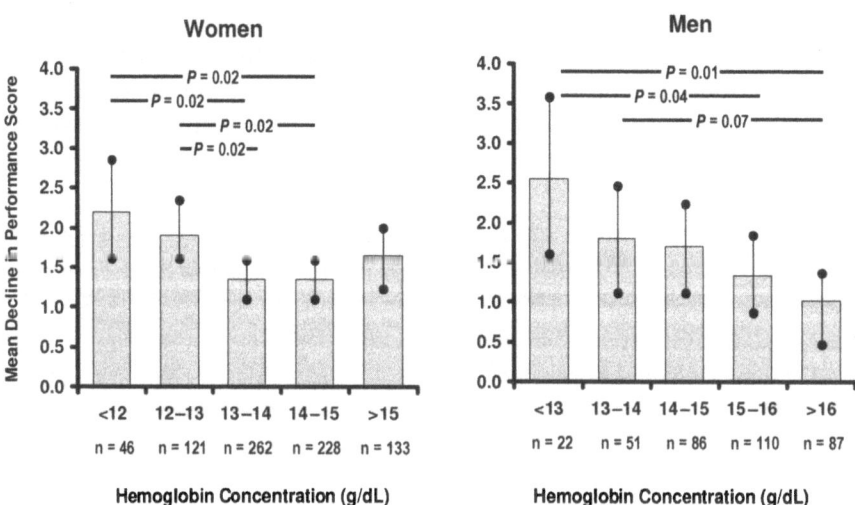

Fig. 10.2 Adjusted mean 4-year decline in physical performance score (1988–1992) in women (left) and men (right) aged 71 years or older as a function of hemoglobin concentration. Decline is adjusted for baseline performance score, age, education, smoking, blood pressure, body mass index, coronary heart disease, heart failure, stroke, diabetes, cancer, infectious disease, and renal disease. *P*-values indicate differences between categories. Vertical lines are 95% confidence intervals (12)

concentrations of 13–15 g/dL. These findings were not changed when subjects who had diseases associated with anemia (eg, CKD, cancer, infections) at baseline or who were hospitalized during the year before baseline were excluded from the analysis (12). Based on these findings, the authors concluded that anemia is a significant and independent risk factor for subsequent physical decline in older men and women.

It has been hypothesized that anemia may also directly affect muscle function. This hypothesis has been directly tested in the InCHIANTI Study, a prospective, population-based study of older people conducted by the Italian National Research Council of Aging (13). InCHIANTI sought to identify risk factors that influence loss of mobility in older adults. Physical performance was assessed with the SPPB in a random sample of 1,008 community-dwelling Italians aged 65–102 (mean age, 75.4 years; 56.1% female). Hand-held dynamometers were used to assess knee extensor strength and hand grip strength. Overall, anemia was present in 11.3% of the participants in the study. Compared with nonanemic subjects, those with anemia were older, had a lower body mass index, and more often had a medical history of heart disease, stroke, gastric ulcer, or renal failure. Physical performance was significantly lower for participants with anemia than for those with normal Hb. Knee extensor strength and hand grip strength were also significantly lower in anemic participants. The findings did not change when persons with iron-deficiency anemia or persons who had been hospitalized in the prior year were excluded from the analysis (13). Subjects with anemia were significantly more likely to report disabilities in basic and instrumental activities of daily life (e.g., eating, bathing, dressing, walking, shopping, doing light housework, etc.) than those with normal Hb, and the number of these disabilities increased as Hb level decreased. Lower limb peripheral quantitative computed tomography of study participants revealed that anemia was not only significantly associated with a lower muscle strength, but also with lower skeletal muscle density and lower fractional muscle area of the calf (14).

So, considering these earlier results, there appears to be evidence that anemia-related impairment of muscle function may exist, which could be due to either direct (e.g., reduced muscle oxygenation or fatigue, weakness) or indirect underlying mechanisms (e.g., through anemia-related inflammation). Since inflammation has negative effects on erythropoiesis and subsequent anemia, inflammation could potentially mediate a link between anemia and physical health decline. In the InChianti study, we explored this potential mediation. While subjects with anemia in this cohort tended to have higher levels of IL-6 and other inflammatory markers (CPR, tumor necrosis factor-α) than those without anemia, addition of IL-6 concentrations as a covariate to the data analysis did not change the significant effect of anemia on physical function measures (13). This suggests that the effect of anemia on physical function exists, rather independent of inflammation. Some other mechanisms could be involved in the anemia-related impairment in function. It could be that reduced muscle oxygenation may result in reduced muscle performance. However, also other potential links between anemia and diminished physical performance cannot be excluded. Anemia may also result in weakness and fatigue, symptoms that could directly reduce physical performance and increase the risk of disability. Also, physical impairment could be secondary to pathophysiological responses to tissue hypoxia resulting from anemia, e.g., myocardial dysfunction, left ventricular hypertrophy (LVH), or reduced blood pressure.

Falls and Fractures

Considering the above described negative effects on muscle and physical performance in persons with anemia, it can be expected that anemia also increases the risk for falling and fall-related fractures. Various study findings do indeed support this expectation. Results from a cross-sectional study of hospital inpatient discharge records for individuals ≥65 years of age obtained from the Wisconsin Bureau of Health Information indicated that 6.9% of 223,085 older adults discharged in 2000 had an unintentional fall. Independent predictors for such falls included age, sex, season of year, area of residence, alcohol-related issues, dementia, Parkinson's disease, mechanical or motor problems, altered consciousness, convulsions/epilepsy, glaucoma, and anemia (15).

Moreover, anemia appears to be associated with increased risk for falls that result in fractures. Retrospective evaluation of 145 patients aged 60–97 years old from nursing homes as well as the community who were hospitalized for hip fracture over a 2-year period indicated that this event was significantly more common in those with anemia (30% vs.. 13%) (16). Analysis of results with a logistic regression model found that anemia was associated with a threefold increase in the risk for falls. Further, each 1 g/dL rise in Hb was associated with a 45% reduction in the risk for falls resulting in fractures (16). Another recent study that evaluated 47,530 elderly subjects (≥65 years of age) included in the Integrated Health Care Information Services national database also indicated that even mild anemia was associated with an increased risk for accidental falls and fractures (17). Most recently, data from a prospective analysis in the Longitudinal Aging Study of Amsterdam population (*n* = 394, age 65–88 years) indicated that WHO-defined anemia was associated with a 91% increased risk for recurrent falls over 3 years of follow-up, and that this relationship was mediated, at least in part, by muscle weakness and poor physical performance in subjects with anemia (18).

Anemia Associated with Cognitive Decline

Cognitive impairment is an extremely common problem in the elderly and an important determinant of elders' ability to function independently. Consequently, cognitive impairment is one of the most important risk factors for disability. Of 536 people ≥65 years of age who were living in the community or in nursing homes, the prevalences of possible cognitive impairment (as assessed by the Mini-Mental State Examination) among anemic and nonanemic men were 55.6 and 34.4%, respectively; and those for anemic and nonanemic women were 47.5 and 40.1% (19). Results from 367 women (70–80 years old) enrolled in the Women's Health and Aging Study II indicated a significant correlation between Hb level and both the Brief Attention and Trail Making B tasks, which are cognitive tests designed to measure attention and executive function performance in an older population. In these older women, lower Hb levels were significantly associated with poorer test performance (20). Finally, results from a recent study from the Gruppo Italiano di Farmacovigilanza nell'Anziano (GIFA) that included 13,301 hospitalized subjects with a mean age of 72 years indicated that participants with cognitive impairment, as defined by a low score on the Abbreviated Mental Test, had a higher risk for WHO-defined anemia (47%) vs. those without cognitive impairment (35%) (21).

Anemia and Consequences of Functional Decline

Earlier paragraphs of this chapter describe various lines of evidence for an unfavorable effect of anemia on indicators of functional health decline (e.g., physical and muscle impairment, cognitive impairment, and disability). Functional health decline increases the risk for general adverse health consequences, such as hospitalizations and mortality. Consequently, partly through its association with functional health decline, it can be hypothesized that anemia also increases the risk for general adverse health outcomes such as hospitalization and mortality. The next paragraphs will describe the results of several studies that have explored these general adverse health outcomes in more detail.

Hospitalization and mortality outcomes were examined prospectively in the EPESE cohort study, a community-based, nationwide study of men and women over 65 years of age in the US. As part of this study, a baseline blood sample was taken from 3,607 participants in 1988, and mortality and hospitalization records were followed for the next 4.5 years (22). The mean age of study participants at baseline was 78.2 years, and the overall prevalence of anemia, as defined by WHO criteria, was 12.5%. Over the 4-year follow-up period, 37% of the persons with anemia vs. 22% of the nonanemic persons died. Compared to subjects who had no anemia, anemic persons had a significantly higher number of hospitalizations (2.0 vs. 1.4), higher number of hospital days (25 vs. 13.7), and the length of stay per hospitalization was significantly longer (10.9 vs. 9.2 days). After adjustment for several baseline and health characteristics, the relative risk of death in anemic persons compared to nonanemic persons was 61% increased, and the corresponding risk for hospitalization was 27% increased. The increased mortality risk extended to persons with Hb levels in the low-normal range (0–1 g/dL above the WHO

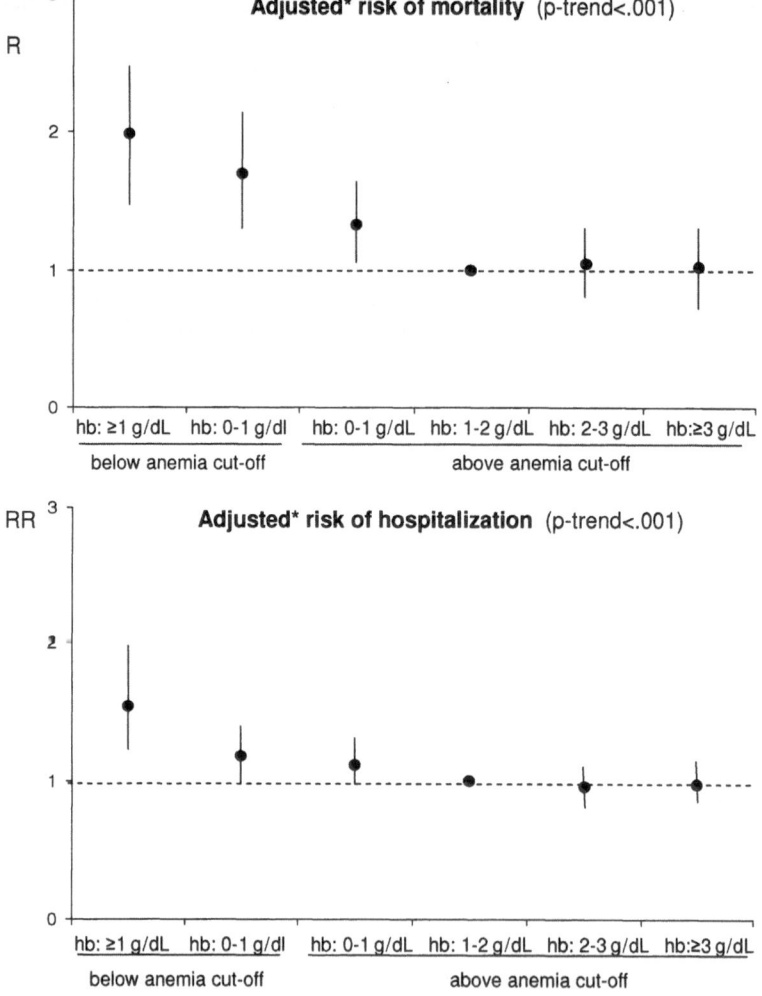

Fig. 10.3. Adjusted* risks of mortality and hospitalization according to hemoglobin level. *Adjusted for age, sex, years of education, smoking, BMI, CHD, CHF, diabetes, cancer, infectious disease, kidney disease, hospitalization in past year. Results from EPESE (22)

threshold) compared with those persons with Hb levels 1–2 g/dL above the anemia cut-off level (see results in Fig. 10.3) (22).

Several other studies have confirmed an association between anemia and increased mortality risk. This relationship was demonstrated in a 10-year community-based study that included 1,016 people ≥85 years of age (23). Compared with subjects with a normal Hb, the mortality risk was 60% increased in anemic women and 130% increased in anemic men. In both sexes, the mortality risk increased with lower Hb concentrations. An assessment of 63 older nursing home residents with Hb < 11 g/dL and age/sex-matched normal controls with Hb ≥ 11 g/dL over a follow-up period of 60 months found that survival was significantly higher in those with high Hb (≥13 mg/dL) (67%) than in those with low Hb (<11 mg/dL) (48%) (24).

Chaves and colleagues assessed the relationship between Hb and 5-year all-cause mortality in 641 community-dwelling women aged ≥65 years of age with moderate-to-severe disability. Results from this study demonstrated a progressive decline in mortality up to an Hb threshold of 13.9 g/dL, which suggests that Hb currently considered as low-normal is associated with a relatively increased mortality risk (25). Most recently, 11.2 years of follow-up of 5,888 community-dwelling men and women ≥65 years age enrolled in the Cardiovascular Health Study indicated a reverse J-shaped relationship between Hb level and mortality. The highest and lowest quintiles of Hb were associated with mortality hazard ratios of 1.33 and 1.17, respectively (26).

Aside from its independent effect on increased mortality in older persons, the presence of anemia as a comorbidity has also been shown to increase mortality in a variety of clinical settings. In a cohort of 12,065 older patients (mean age approximately 77 years) with new-onset congestive heart failure (CHF), 17% were found to have anemia (27). In a subsequent 5-year follow-up, CHF patients with anemia were found to have an adjusted relative risk of mortality of 1.34 (95% CI: 1.24–1.46) compared to CHF patients without anemia, indicating that anemia is an independent prognostic factor for mortality in CHF patients. The investigators speculated that correction of anemia might improve the prognosis of CHF patients.

Anemia is also a risk factor in older patients with a recent myocardial infarction (MI). In a retrospective study, 78,974 Medicare patients aged 65 years or older were categorized by hematocrit (Hct) upon admission after an acute MI and followed for outcomes (28). An inverse relationship between admission Hct and mortality was noted. Even modest anemia, Hct ~ 33%, was associated with a near doubling of the risk of short-term death. Treatment of patients with Hct of 33% or lower with blood transfusion was associated with a reduction in risk of 30-day mortality. In a more stable population of elderly patients with compensated CHF, Silverberg and colleagues (29) found anemia to be an independent predictor of increased mortality. Recent results from the Evaluation of Losartan In The Elderly (ELITE II) trial indicated that anemia was a significant independent predictor of mortality in patients with CHF (30). Finally, a prospective analysis of 225 elective total hip replacements indicated that patients with preclinical anemia at the time of admission had higher incidences of postoperative infection and transfusion and longer postoperative inpatient stays (31).

Summary and Implications

In the community-dwelling older population at large, anemia is a common clinical syndrome, and predominantly mild. Several observational data from large, community-based studies have consistently shown independent associations of mild anemia with major adverse outcomes in older adults, such as decline in physical function, disability, falls, cognitive decline, hospitalization, and mortality. Results of several studies suggest that the deleterious effects of anemia may occur at Hb concentrations that typically have been considered low normal by current WHO standards. This has been supported by physiological data showing optimally lowest levels of serum erythropoietin, a surrogate marker of tissue hypoxemia, around WHO mid-normal levels (32). It must be acknowledged, though, that what may seem optimal Hb from the perspective of lowest risk of adverse outcomes, may not be optimal for screening purposes, given that the latter should aim at maximizing potential clinical benefits, while minimizing the burden associated with additional investigation of anemia. In addition, little is known about whether Hb thresholds for the definition of anemia in older adults should vary or not according to gender, race, and health status.

In regards to the nature of the associations between anemia and functional health decline and related adverse clinical outcomes; i.e., causal vs. noncausal, it remains to be ultimately determined, as independent associations in observational studies are not necessarily causal. Such a determination is critical vis-à-vis understanding opportunities for intervention. A major hypothesis is that even mild reductions in Hb could lead to diminished delivery of oxygen to the tissues, with consequent decrease in exercise-tolerance and muscle strength mass, further deconditioning, and ultimately disability. Indirectly, anemia reflects the presence of major chronic diseases and inflammation, both of which are independently related to disability and mortality. Even though most studies adequately took comorbidities into account, it cannot be excluded that anemia partly reflects disease severity or subclinical disease states resulting in physical decline. On-going research effort is anticipated to contribute to a better understanding about the physiological mechanisms underlying the adverse functional health consequences of late-life anemia. In addition, assessments of the need and efficacy of therapy for mild anemia in older adults vis-à-vis preventing and/or ameliorating adverse outcomes such as disability are warranted in the future.

References

1. Verbrugge LM, Jette AM. The disablement process. *Soc Sci Med.* 1994;38:1–14.
2. World Health Organization. International classification of functioning, disability and health. 2001. Geneva, Switzerland, WHO.
3. Kramarow E, Lentzner H, Rooks R, Weeks J, Saydah S. Health and Aging Chartbook. Health, United States, 1999. Hyattsville, MD, National Center for Health Statistics.
4. Guralnik JM, Ferrucci L, Simonsick EM, Salive ME, Wallace RB. Lower-extremity function in persons over the age of 70 years as a predictor of subsequent disability. *N Engl J Med.* 1995;332:556–561.
5. Penninx BW, Ferrucci L, Leveille SG, Rantanen T, Pahor M, Guralnik JM. Lower extremity performance in nondisabled older persons as a predictor of subsequent hospitalization. *J Gerontol A Biol Sci Med Sci.* 2000;55:M691–M697.
6. Guralnik JM, Fried LP, Salive ME. Disability as a public health outcome in the aging population. *Annu Rev Public Health.* 1996;17:25–46.
7. Fried TR, Bradley EH, Williams CS, Tinetti ME. Functional disability and health care expenditures for older persons. *Arch Intern Med.* 2001;161:2602–2607.
8. Chaves PH, Ashar B, Guralnik JM, Fried LP. Looking at the relationship between hemoglobin concentration and prevalent mobility difficulty in older women. Should the criteria currently used to define anemia in older people be reevaluated? *J Am Geriatr Soc.* 2002;50:1257–1264.
9. Guralnik JM, Simonsick EM, Ferrucci L, et al. A short physical performance battery assessing lower extremity function: association with self-reported disability and prediction of mortality and nursing home admission. *J Gerontol.* 1994;49:M85–M94.
10. Penninx BW, Ferrucci L, Leveille SG, Rantanen T, Pahor M, Guralnik JM. Lower extremity performance in nondisabled older persons as a predictor of subsequent hospitalization. *J Gerontol A Biol Sci Med Sci.* 2000;55:M691–M697.
11. Guralnik JM, Winograd CH. Physical performance measures in the assessment of older persons. *Aging (Milano).* 1994;6:303–305.
12. Penninx BW, Guralnik JM, Onder G, Ferrucci L, Wallace RB, Pahor M. Anemia and decline in physical performance among older persons. *Am J Med.* 2003;115:104–110.
13. Penninx BW, Pahor M, Cesari M, et al. Anemia is associated with disability and decreased physical performance and muscle strength in the elderly. *J Am Geriatr Soc.* 2004;52:719–724.
14. Cesari M, Penninx BW, Lauretani F, Russo CR, Carter C, Bandinelli S, Atkinson H, Onder G, Pahor M, Ferrucci L. Hemoglobin levels and skeletal muscle: results from the InCHIANTI study. *J Gerontol A Biol Sci Med Sci.* 2004;59:249–254.
15. Guse CE, Porinsky R. Risk factors associated with hospitalization for unintentional falls: Wisconsin hospital discharge data for patients aged 65 and over. *WMJ.* 2003;102:37–42.

16. Dharmarajan TS, Avula S, Norkus EP. Anemia increases risk for falls in hospitalized older adults: an evaluation of falls in 362 hospitalized, ambulatory, long-term care, and community patients. *J Am Med Dir Assoc*. 2006;7:287–293.

17. Duh MS, Lefebvre P, Buteau S, Mody SH, Woodman R. Anemia and risk of accidental falls/fractures in the elderly. *J Am Geriatr Soc*. 2005;53 (Suppl 4):S8–S83.

18. Penninx BW, Pluijm SM, Lips P, et al. Late-life anemia is associated with increased risk of recurrent falls. *J Am Geriatr Soc*. 2005;53:2106–2111.

19. Argyriadou S, Vlachonikolis I, Melisopoulou H, Katachanakis K, Lionis C. In what extent anemia coexists with cognitive impairment in elderly: a cross-sectional study in Greece. *BMC Fam Pract*. 2001;2:5.

20. Chaves PH, Carlson MC, Ferrucci L, Guralnik JM, Semba R, Fried LP. Association between mild anemia and executive function impairment in community-dwelling older women: The Women's Health and Aging Study II. *J Am Geriatr Soc*. 2006;54:1429–1435.

21. Zamboni V, Cesari M, Zuccala G, et al. Anemia and cognitive performance in hospitalized older patients: results from the GIFA study. *Int J Geriatr Psychiatry*. 2006;21:529–534.

22. Penninx BW, Pahor M, Woodman RC, Guralnik JM. Anemia in old age is associated with increased mortality and hospitalization. *J Gerontol A Biol Sci Med Sci*. 2006;61:474–479.

23. Izaks GJ, Westendorp RG, Knook DL. The definition of anemia in older persons. *JAMA*. 1999;281:1714–1717.

24. Kikuchi M, Inagaki T, Shinagawa N. Five-year survival of older people with anemia: variation with hemoglobin concentration. *J Am Geriatr Soc*. 2001;49:1226–1228.

25. Chaves PH, Xue QL, Guralnik JM, Ferrucci L, Volpato S, Fried LP. What constitutes normal hemoglobin concentration in community-dwelling disabled older women? *J Am Geriatr Soc*. 2004;52:1811–1816.

26. Zakai NA, Katz R, Hirsch C, et al. A prospective study of anemia status, hemoglobin concentration, and mortality in an elderly cohort: the Cardiovascular Health Study. *Arch Intern Med*. 2005;165:2214–2220.

27. Ezekowitz JA, McAlister FA, Armstrong PW. Anemia is common in heart failure and is associated with poor outcomes: insights from a cohort of 12 065 patients with new-onset heart failure. *Circulation*. 2003;107:223–225.

28. Wu WC, Rathore SS, Wang Y, Radford MJ, Krumholz HM. Blood transfusion in elderly patients with acute myocardial infarction. *N Engl J Med*. 2001;345:1230–1236.

29. Silverberg DS, Wexler D, Iaina A. The role of anemia in the progression of congestive heart failure. Is there a place for erythropoietin and intravenous iron? *J Nephrol*. 2004;17:749–761.

30. Sharma R, Francis DP, Pitt B, Poole-Wilson PA, Coats AJ, Anker SD. Haemoglobin predicts survival in patients with chronic heart failure: a substudy of the ELITE II trial. *Eur Heart J*. 2004;25:1021–1028.

31. Myers E, Grady PO, Dolan AM. The influence of preclinical anaemia on outcome following total hip replacement. *Arch Orthop Trauma Surg*. 2004;124:699–701.

32. Ferrucci L, Guralnik JM, Woodman RC, Bandinelli S, Lauretani F, Corsi AM, et al. Proinflammatory state and circulating erythropoietin in persons with and without anemia. *Am J Med* 2005;118:1288–1296.

Subject Index